Opposition in Pilates and Yoga

A conceptual blend of Newton's
Third Law and mindfulness

MARIE-CLAIRE PRETTYMAN

Opposition in Pilates and Yoga

First published in 2016 by

Panoma Press Ltd
48 St Vincent Drive, St Albans, Herts, AL1 5SJ, UK

info@panomapress.com
www.panomapress.com

Book design and layout by Neil Coe.

Printed on acid-free paper from managed forests.

ISBN 978-1-784520-76-2

Dedication

This book is for everyone I have ever had the pleasure of teaching – both clients and trainee teachers alike.

And it is for everyone with whom I have yet to work.

In memory of my beautiful colleague Heidi Lacey and my funny and brave client Heather Quinn.

I hope this makes you proud ladies…

Acknowledgments

Katey Fox you are both a great friend and a hugely talented photographer. It has been so much fun working with you. Thank you for all of your efforts. Looking forward to next time!

www.kateyfoxphotography.co.uk

Contents

How to use this guide

Are you familiar with Newton's Third Law? It states that:

For every action, there is an equal and opposite reaction.

This got me thinking. In movement, if we want to lift a part of the body, there must be another part of the body that has to drop down. If we stretch away with one limb, we need to stretch away in the opposite direction with another limb (at the other end of the body).

I experimented with this for some time in classes and with private clients and found that not only does this way of approach to movement help participants understand what is required of them in terms of the execution, it also naturally creates work in the appropriate muscles!

'Appropriate muscles' is key here. We all have different postures depending on our habits, sports and genetics. One person may have an anteriorly (forward) tilting pelvis and another a posterior (backward) tilting pelvis. Immediately, they are opposite in terms of their muscle lengths and strengths on each side of the body. This means that they will feel muscles work potentially in different places in the same exercise or posture. This does not mean that one is right and the other is wrong, merely that they have different needs, different strengths, different weaknesses.

I have read countless books about Pilates and Yoga and many of them dictate where you should feel the work. They do not account for individual differences, and assume that everyone is perfect so therefore everyone will feel the exercise or posture in the same place in the same way.

This guide strips away the assumption that everybody is put together in exactly the same way and accounts for individuality by using Newton's principles and MINDFULNESS to keep the body safe in movement and allow YOU to feel whatever it is you need to feel, or work whatever it is you need to work.

The exercise pages are designed in such a way that if you do not want to, you do not need to read the text below unless you feel you must, to increase understanding. The arrows show a direction of 'energy'. Predominantly UP and DOWN, but sometimes you will see either a left or right arrow, or both. These will be explained using the sub-heading OTHER (energy). The arrows demonstrate the need to create opposite forces by focusing your attention on the direction they show. This is 'opposition', and the cornerstone of this book. This is not an exact science; sometimes there may be a directional arrow without an opposite. Remember, this is a concept designed to de-mystify the art of movement.

Unless identified as Advanced, all the exercises or postures are suitable for all levels – Beginners, Intermediate and Advanced. If an exercise or posture has a number of stages of difficulty, you will see a number next to the title e.g. **Hamstring Stretch 1**. As a beginner, please choose 1 until your body is comfortable with the exercise or posture. **Please do not move on until your body is ready.**

To create *opposition*, you need to concentrate and be aware of your body, be 'mindful'. The concept of mindfulness is well understood in terms of stress relief and the management of anxiety and depression. We are going to explore mindfulness in movement, listening to your body and allowing it to exist comfortably within its natural parameters. Accepting the limitations it imposes on you as well as appreciating the progressions you will make.

Mindfulness

Mindfulness is the gentle effort to be continuously present with experience.

or

'Mindfulness means paying attention in a particular way, on purpose, in the present moment, and nonjudgmentally.'

Jon Kabat-Zinn

Kabat-Zinn is a famous teacher of mindfulness meditation and the founder of the 'Mindfulness-Based Stress Reduction' program at the University of Massachusetts Medical Center.

Paying attention 'on purpose'

First of all, mindfulness involves paying attention 'on purpose'. Mindfulness involves a conscious direction of our awareness. We sometimes talk about 'mindfulness' and 'awareness' as if they were interchangeable terms, but that's not a good habit to get into. I may be aware that I'm irritable, but that wouldn't mean I was being mindful of my irritability. In order to be mindful, I have to be purposefully aware of myself, not just vaguely and habitually aware. Knowing that you are eating is not the same as eating mindfully.

Let's take that example of eating and look at it a bit further. When we are purposefully aware of eating, we are consciously being aware of the process of eating. We're deliberately noticing the sensations and our responses to those sensations. We're noticing the mind wandering, and when it does wander we purposefully bring our attention back.

When we're eating 'unmindfully' we may in theory be aware of what we're doing, but we're probably thinking about a hundred and one other things at the same time, and we may also be watching TV, talking, or reading, or even all three! So a very small part of our awareness is absorbed with eating and we may be only barely aware of the physical sensations, and even less aware of our thoughts and emotions.

Because we're only dimly aware of our thoughts, they wander in an unrestricted way. There's no conscious attempt to bring our attention back to our eating. There's no purposefulness.

This purposefulness is a very important part of mindfulness.

Having the purpose of staying with our experience, whether that's the breath, or a particular emotion, a movement, or something as simple as eating, means that we are actively shaping the mind.

Paying attention 'in the present moment'

Left to itself the mind wanders through all kinds of thoughts, including thoughts expressing anger, craving, depression, revenge, self-pity, etc. As we indulge in these kinds of thoughts we reinforce those emotions in our hearts and cause ourselves to suffer. Mostly these thoughts are about the past or future. The past no longer exists and the future is just a fantasy until it happens. The one moment we actually can experience, the present moment, is the one we seem to most avoid.

So in mindfulness we're concerned with noticing what's going on right now. That doesn't mean we can no longer think about the past or future, but when we do so, we do so mindfully, so that we're aware that right now we're thinking about the past or future.

However, in meditation we are concerned with what's arising in the present moment. When thoughts about the past or future take us away from our present moment experience and we 'space out', we try to notice this and just come back to now.

By purposefully directing our awareness away from such thoughts and toward the 'anchor' of our present moment experience, we decrease their effect on our lives and we create instead a space of freedom where calmness and contentment can grow.

Paying attention 'non-judgmentally'

Mindfulness is an emotionally non-reactive state. We don't judge that this experience is good and that one is bad. Or if we do make those judgments we simply notice them and let go of them. We don't get upset because we're experiencing something we don't want to be experiencing or because we're not experiencing what we would rather be experiencing. We simply accept whatever arises. We observe it mindfully. We notice it arising, passing through us, and ceasing to exist.

Whether it's a pleasant experience or a painful experience we treat it the same way.

Cognitively, mindfulness is aware that certain experiences are pleasant and some are unpleasant, but on an emotional level we simply don't react. We call this 'equanimity' – stillness and balance of mind.

Mindfulness and movement

Consider for a moment how it feels to stand up. You stand up every day: you stand at work, you stand while you talk to people, you stand in the checkout at the supermarket. You do not have to think about HOW you are standing, you just are. To get the best from this guide, you need to consider every moment that you are moving in an exercise and holding a posture. You must start to think about what your body is doing 'on purpose', be 'in the present' to understand what you are feeling in your body and appreciate the activity. Try not to judge your perceived 'ability'. Work with your own body, in its own unique state, and soon it will start to work more efficiently for you and you will feel the benefits, both in body and mind.

Neutral Pelvis and Neutral Spine

Before you continue with the guide, it is important to consider the foundation on which you are going to move.

A strong base of support will dictate the efficiency of the movement or posture.

A Neutral Pelvis and Neutral Spine, simply put, means having both of those parts of the body sitting in their most biomechanically efficient positions.

Consider:

The Pelvis

Each half of the pelvic girdle is made of the:

Ilium
Ischium
&
Pubis

These bones are bound together and the two halves bound together:

Anteriorly at the pubic symphysis
&
Posteriorly with the sacrum and coccyx via the sacroiliac joints

The pubic symphysis and the sacroiliac joints are held together with strong ligaments and have relatively little movement.

The position of the pelvis in relation to the spine

Think of the effects of the position of the pelvis in relation to the spine. The fifth lumbar vertebra rests upon the slanted sacral table, producing *intrinsic shear forces* in the lower lumbar area.

An excessive forward tilt (**anterior**) of the top of the pelvis increases the lumbosacral angle deepening the lumbar curve, which increases the other spinal curves. It means that the vertebrae are not aligned well on top of each other, increasing the shear stresses.

If the pelvis is tilted or rotated, the spine will compensate accordingly.

If the pelvic crests are not level in the horizontal plane, the lumbar spine will deviate to the lower side of the pelvis. This will force the spine into a corrective curve to regain its vertical alignment. If the pelvic halves are twisted, the spine may twist uncomfortably at its base.

An excessive backward (**posterior**) tilt of the pelvis will flatten the curves and the spine will lose its shock-absorbing ability. The muscle balance is also upset, particularly the function of iliopsoas, so hip flexion and extension will be restricted.

The pelvis may be tilted or twisted due to various factors. True leg length differences are not very common. Muscle imbalance is the most common cause.

The pelvis needs to be stable and in its neutral position so there is no strain on its joints.

In order to be biomechanically efficient, we must position the pelvis in between the two excessive positions. Not anterior, with an excessive curve in the lower back, or posterior, with a flattened lower back.

When you lie in **The Relaxation Position**, the hip bones and the pubic bone should be level, as if you were going to place a tray across them.

The spine should exist with its natural curves, about a flat hand's width between the lower back and the floor, all of the ribcage down into the floor and a gentle curve in the neck so that the face is parallel to the floor and ceiling; a thin pillow may help with that.

Try to maintain this concept of Neutral Pelvis and Neutral Spine as you work your way through the guide.

Breathing

Please try not to **fixate** on the breathing. Breathing is innate, it is fundamentally human. As long as you remember to just keep breathing, the 'correct' way will develop naturally.

Pilates and Yoga breathing differs in one key area, where we send the breath into the body. In Pilates, we aim to maintain a strong center i.e. the abdominals remain contracted throughout the exercises. We cannot breathe abdominally in Pilates because we would lose the connection between the ribcage and the pelvis. Therefore, we aim to send the breath wide into the ribcage and into the back of the body.

When you start Pilates your intercostal muscles may by tight and unyielding to this kind of breath work. If you make too much effort to breathe in this way, you may find that you do not have the space in your ribcage to take a full inhale. It is better to allow your muscles to stretch gently, the ribcage to become more mobile, and the abdominals to develop strength gradually, rather than forcing it. Breathe comfortably, just know in your mind what the aim is as you improve.

Yoga is different; in this practice we aim to send the breath into the abdomen. The belly expands as we inhale and retracts as we exhale. You can see that this type of breath work is not appropriate for Pilates exercises, but in Yoga it can provide a deeper sense of stillness and awareness in postures. It encourages us to receive as much oxygen as we can from the inhalation and expel as much carbon dioxide as we can during the exhalation. Be careful with this type of breath work when you start; the increased inhalation can lead to oxygen saturation in the bloodstream, which can cause dizziness.

As you get used to the exercises and postures, you will find the breathing evolves in an organic way. It will feel natural to breathe in a certain way. When you start, just enjoy moving and breathe in a way that feels natural to you, just *avoid holding your breath.*

Interestingly, holding the breath is a fundamental practice in yoga. It creates stillness again in body and mind. Breath holding is also used in meditation practices for the same reason. However, I would not recommend it as you work your way through this guide.

A Final Note

Concentrate, be mindful, listen to your body
and follow the guide.

You are aiming to repeat each **Pilates** exercise
eight times unless otherwise stated.

If directed to 'hold' a **Yoga** posture,
I recommend three breath cycles.

If you are unsure about breath patterns,
simply *breathe comfortably* until you are more
familiar with your routine/practice.

Pilates

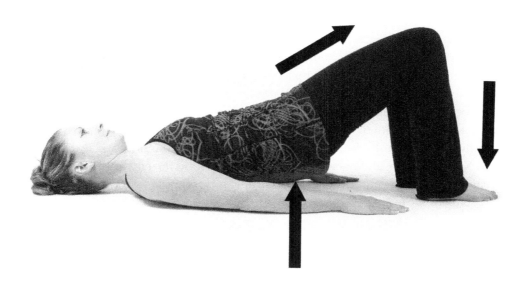

The Relaxation Position

AIM: To relax the muscles and re-establish the efficient flow of cerebrospinal fluid.

Opposition:

↑ UP: Create a sense of lightness at the knees, which will also create a sense of heaviness at the pelvis (*opposition*).

↓ DOWN: Maintain a positive connection between the ribcage, pelvis and the floor.

Directions:

Lie on your back with your knees bent and your pelvis and spine in a neutral position (see pages 11 & 12). Position your arms by the sides of your body, palms down if that is comfortable for you, palms up if not. Allow your body to settle into the floor. Relax the shoulders so that the collarbones widen, and lengthen the back of the neck. Focus on sending the **inhale** into the back and sides of your ribcage, so that it does not lift the bottom of the ribcage up. Keep the muscles of the abdomen drawn in gently. As you **exhale**, feel the ribcage drawing in from the sides and down at the front. Notice how the abdomen naturally draws in toward the end of the exhale. Try to maintain the connection at your abdomen as you continue to inhale and exhale.

Other considerations:

You may feel more comfortable with a small pillow under your head; this will help with the ribcage connection.

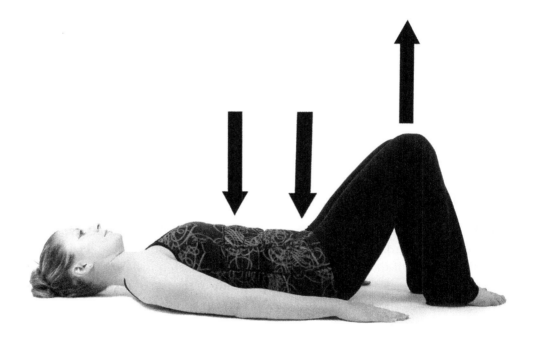

Single Knee Fold

AIM: To strengthen the lower abdominals and maintain the integrity between the ribcage and the pelvis, and to increase the stability of the pelvis.

Opposition:

↑ UP: Create a sense of lightness under your feet, which gradually increases in order to float the leg away from the floor.

↓ DOWN: Maintain a strong connection between the ribcage and the floor. Allow the pelvis to sink more heavily into the floor, *in opposition*.

Directions:

Inhale into the back and sides of the ribcage to prepare. As you **exhale**, focus on the *opposition*. Toward the end of the exhale, you should feel able to float the leg away from the floor until the thigh bone is vertical and the shin is horizontal. You will notice the abdominals working throughout. **Inhale** at the top of the range. **Exhale** until you feel the abdominals tightening, then start to lower the leg, focusing on heaviness of the pelvis.

Other considerations:

Maintain a positive connection between the ribcage and the floor. Avoid gripping in the 'non-working' leg.

Keep the shoulders relaxed.

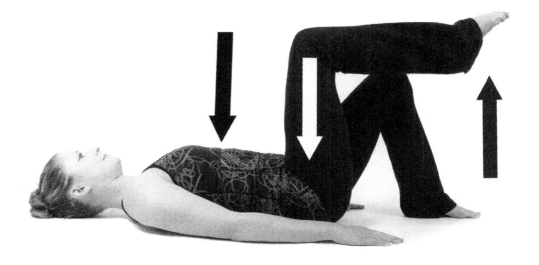

Double Knee Fold

AIM: To further strengthen the lower abdominals and maintain the integrity between the ribcage and the pelvis, and to increase the stability of the pelvis.

Opposition:

↑ UP: Create a sense of lightness under your feet, which gradually increases in order to float the leg away from the floor.

↓ DOWN: Maintain a positive connection between the ribcage and the floor. Allow the pelvis to sink more heavily into the floor, *in opposition* to the lifting leg(s).

Directions:

Inhale into the back and sides of the ribcage to prepare. As you **exhale**, focus on the *opposition* (light feet, heavy pelvis, heavy ribcage). Toward the end of the exhale, you should feel able to float the leg away from the floor until the thigh bone is vertical and the shin is horizontal. You will notice the abdominals working throughout. Repeat with the other leg, being careful to avoid arching the back or 'doming' the abdominals. **Inhale** at the top of the range. **Exhale** until you feel the abdominals tightening again, then start to lower one leg at a time, focusing on the heaviness of the pelvis.

Other considerations:

Avoid gripping in the 'non-working' leg.

Keep the shoulders relaxed.

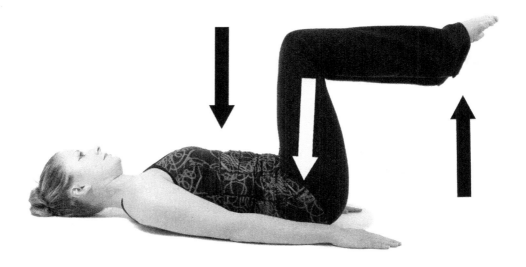

Toe Taps 1

AIM: To further strengthen the lower abdominals and maintain the integrity between the ribcage and the pelvis, and to increase the stability of the pelvis.

Opposition:

↑ UP: Maintain the sense of lightness under your feet.

↓ DOWN: Maintain a positive connection between the ribcage and the floor. Allow the pelvis to sink more heavily into the floor, *in opposition* to the lowering leg(s).

Directions:

Inhale into the back and sides of the ribcage to prepare. As you **exhale**, focus on the *opposition* (heavy pelvis, heavy ribcage, light feet) and start to lower one set of toes toward the floor. You will notice the abdominal work increasing as the foot lowers. After touching the toes down, **inhale** and lift the leg back up. Repeat with the other leg.

Other considerations:

Avoid arching the back and allowing the abdominals to 'dome' throughout the exercise. Avoid gripping in the 'non-working' leg.

Keep the shoulders relaxed and the spine long.

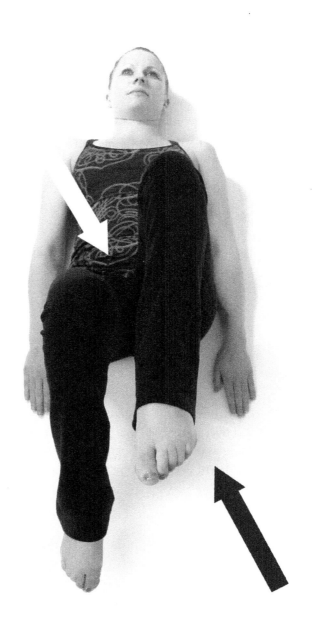

The Dying Bug / Toe Taps 2

AIM: To further strengthen the lower abdominals and establish a stronger connection between the ribcage and the pelvis. To increase the stability of the pelvis and the stability of the shoulders.

Opposition:

↑ UP: Maintain the sense of lightness under your feet.

↓ DOWN: Increase the connection between the ribcage and the floor. Allow the pelvis to sink more heavily into the floor, in *opposition* to the lowering leg(s).

Directions:

Inhale into the back and sides of the ribcage to prepare. As you **exhale**, focus on the *opposition* (heavy pelvis, heavy ribcage, light feet) and start to lower one set of toes toward the floor and take the opposite arm over your head. You will notice the abdominal work increasing as the foot and arm lower. After touching the toes down, **inhale** and lift the leg and arm back up. Repeat with the other side.

Other considerations:

Keep the arm in your peripheral vision at the end of the range to avoid shoulder displacement and arching of the back. Avoid 'doming' the abdominals.

Keep the spine long and the shoulders relaxed.

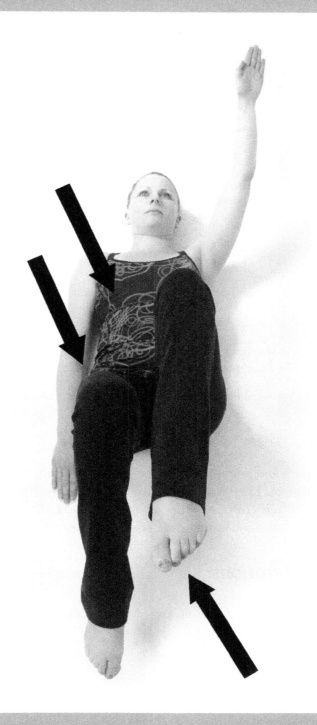

Spine Curls

AIM: To articulate the spine and strengthen the buttocks while lengthening the hip flexors.

Opposition:

↑ UP: 1. Create a sense of lightness at the knees.

2. Squeeze the buttocks to lift.

↓ DOWN: 1 & 2. Maintain a balanced and positive connection between the feet and the floor, particularly the base of the big toe.

OTHER (energy): Lengthen the knees away from you as you lift.

Directions:

Inhale to the back and sides of the ribcage to prepare. **Exhale** and roll the pelvis until the back flattens. Keep rolling and lifting the spine one bone at a time for the duration of the exhale. **Inhale** at the top of the range. **Exhale** and roll the spine back down to the relaxation position one bone at a time.

Other considerations:

Avoid lifting the ribcage as you lift up and keep the back of the neck long.

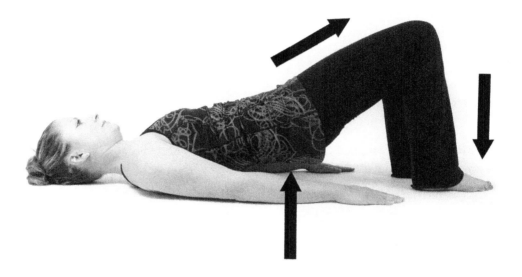

Spine Curls with Arms

AIM: To further challenge the connection between the ribcage and the pelvis. To work the shoulder stabilizers.

Opposition:

↑ UP: Squeeze the buttocks to lift.

↓ DOWN: Maintain a balanced and positive connection between the feet and the floor, particularly the base of the big toe.

OTHER (energy): Lengthen the knees away from you as you lift and the arms away from you as you lower.

Directions:

Inhale to the back and sides of the ribcage to prepare. **Exhale** and roll the pelvis until the back flattens. Keep rolling and lifting the spine one bone at a time for the duration of the exhale. **Inhale** at the top of the range and take both arms over the head. **Exhale** and roll the spine back down to the relaxation position one bone at a time, leaving the arms over your head. **Inhale** to return the arms to your sides.

Other considerations:

Avoid lifting the ribcage as you lift up and lower and keep the back of the neck long.

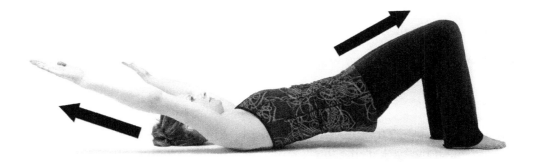

Hamstring Stretch 1

AIM: To stretch/lengthen the hamstrings.

Opposition:

↑ **UP:**   Lengthen out through the toes.

↓ **DOWN:**   Allow the pelvis to drop heavily into the floor.

Directions:

Position yourself in **The Relaxation Position**. **Single Knee Fold** one leg up and reach behind the back of the thigh, lacing your fingers together. Stretch the leg up to a point where you feel a stretch and hold it. Breathe in a relaxed manner until the stretch is less intense.

Other considerations:

Maintain a positive connection between the ribcage and the floor. Keep the shoulders relaxed and the back of the neck long. Avoid gripping in the 'non-working' leg. Keep the other foot balanced, particularly paying attention to the base of the big toe.

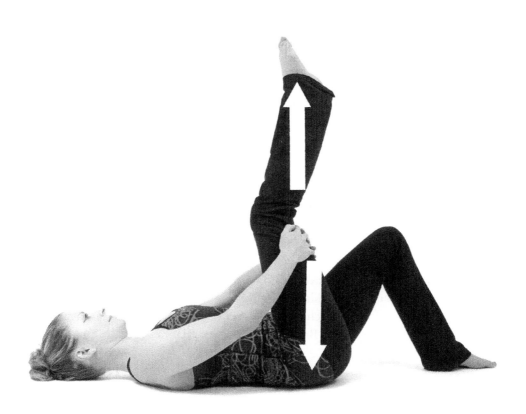

Hamstring Stretch 2

AIM: To stretch/lengthen the hamstrings.

Opposition:

↑ UP: Lengthen out through the toes.

↓ DOWN: Allow the pelvis to drop heavily into the floor.

Directions:

Position yourself in **The Relaxation Position**. **Single Knee Fold** one leg up and reach behind the back of the thigh, lacing your fingers together. Stretch the leg up to a point where you feel a stretch and hold it. Slide the other leg out along the floor, keeping the knee slightly bent. Breathe in a relaxed manner until the stretch is less intense.

Other considerations:

Maintain a positive connection between the ribcage and the floor. Keep the shoulders relaxed and the back of the neck long. Avoid gripping in the 'non-working' leg. Turn the foot out from the ankle on the 'non-working' leg.

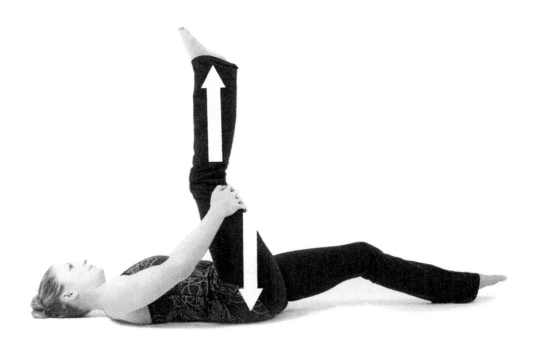

Hamstring Stretch 3

(Advanced)

AIM: To stretch the hamstrings.

Opposition:

↑ UP: Lengthen out through the toes.

↓ DOWN: Allow the pelvis to drop heavily into the floor.

OTHER (energy): Stretch the non-working leg out along the floor *in opposition* to the other leg.

Directions:

Lie in **The Relaxation Position. Single Knee Fold** one leg up and reach behind the back of the thigh, lacing your fingers together. Stretch the leg up to a point where you feel a stretch and hold it. Slide the other leg out along the floor until the leg is straight and turned out at the foot. Breathe in a relaxed manner until the stretch is less intense.

Other considerations:

Maintain a positive connection between the ribcage and the floor. Keep the shoulders relaxed and the back of the neck long.

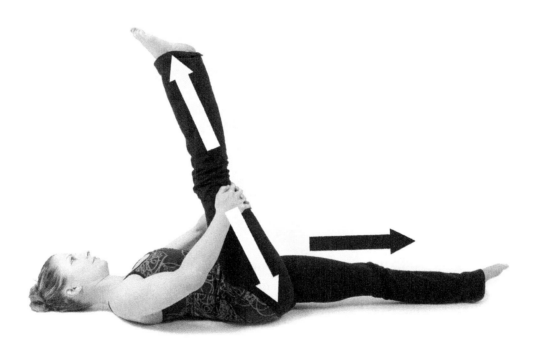

Curl Up 1

AIM: To strengthen the abdominals.

Opposition:

↑ UP: 1. Create a sense of lightness at the knees and maintain it.

2. When you lift, lengthen out through the elbows and the top of the head. The feet will feel light at the top of the movement.

↓ DOWN: 1 & 2. Maintain a positive connection between the ribcage and the floor. Allow the pelvis to drop heavily into the floor, *in opposition* to the lift of the upper body and the lightness of the feet.

Directions:

Position yourself in **The Relaxation Position** and lace your fingers together around the back of your head.* **Inhale** into the back and sides of your ribcage to prepare. As you **exhale**, lift the upper body up away from the floor, the pelvis will become heavier. Draw in through the abdominals. **Inhale** into the back and sides of the ribcage to create more lift (without force). **Exhale** and return to the start.

Other considerations:

Keep the abdominals drawn in throughout.

Keep the weight of your head heavy in your hands. This is extremely important to prevent neck strain.

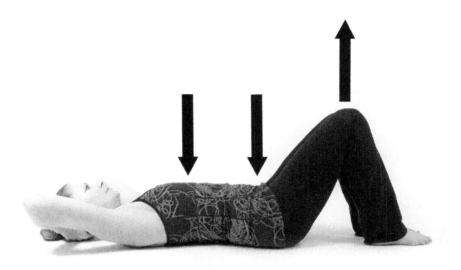

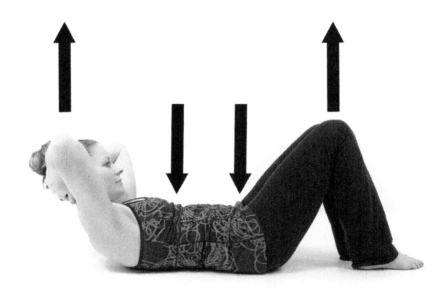

Curl Up 2
(with Single Knee Fold)

AIM: To strengthen the abdominals and improve pelvic stability.

Opposition:

↑ UP: Create a sense of lightness at the knees and maintain it. When you lift, lengthen out through the elbows and the top of the head. The feet will feel light at the top of the movement.

↓ DOWN: Maintain a positive connection between the ribcage and the floor. Allow the pelvis to drop heavily into the floor, *in opposition* to the lift of the upper body and lift of the leg.

Directions:

Position yourself in **The Relaxation Position** and lace your fingers together around the back of your head.* **Inhale** into the back and sides of your ribcage to prepare. As you **exhale**, lift the upper body up away from the floor, the pelvis will become heavier. Allow one foot to become lighter until you can float it away from the floor. Keep the abdominals drawn in. **Inhale** into the back and sides of the ribcage to create more lift (without force). **Exhale** and return to the start.

Other considerations:

Keep the abdominals drawn in throughout. Maintain a 90 degree angle under the knees.

*Keep the weight of your head heavy in your hands. This is extremely important to prevent neck strain.

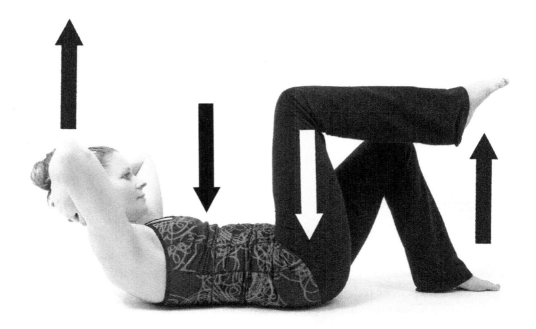

Curl Up 3
(with Double Knee Fold) (Advanced)

AIM: To strengthen the abdominals and further improve pelvic stability.

Opposition:

↑ UP: Create a sense of lightness at the knees and maintain it. When you lift, lengthen out through the elbows and the top of the head. The feet will feel light at the top of the movement.

↓ DOWN: Maintain a positive connection between the ribcage and the floor. Allow the pelvis to drop heavily into the floor, *in opposition* to the lift of the upper body and the lightness of the feet.

Directions:

Position yourself in **The Relaxation Position** and lace your fingers together around the back of your head.* **Inhale** into the back and sides of your ribcage to prepare. As you **exhale**, lift the upper body up away from the floor, the pelvis will become heavier. Allow one foot to become lighter until you can float it away from the floor. Follow with the other leg. Keep the abdominals drawn in. **Inhale** into the back and sides of the ribcage to create more lift (without force). **Exhale** and return to the start, lowering one leg at a time.

Other considerations:

Keep the abdominals drawn in throughout. Maintain a 90 degree angle under the knees.

Keep the weight of your head heavy in your hands. This is extremely important to prevent neck strain.

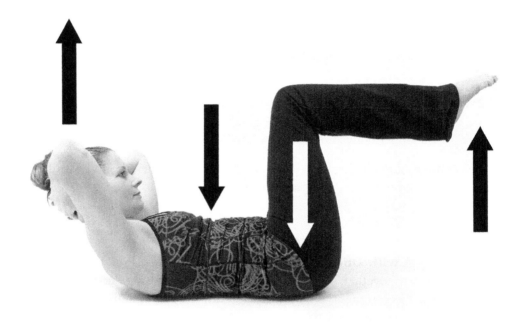

One Hundred 1

AIM: To strengthen the abdominals and increase the heart rate.

Opposition:

↑ UP: Create a sense of lightness under the feet and lengthen out through the top of the head.

↓ DOWN: Maintain a positive connection between the ribcage and the floor. Allow the pelvis to drop heavily into the floor, *in opposition* to the lift of the upper body and the lightness of the feet.

OTHER (energy): Send the arms away from you alongside the body with the shoulders back and the fingers long and strong.

Directions:

From **Curl Up 3 with Double Knee Fold,** stretch the arms out alongside the body. Bring the legs together, keeping them at 90 degrees. **Inhale** and **exhale** fully for a count of 10 as you pump the arms up and down vigorously, from in line with the body to slightly above and back again.*

Other considerations:

Keep the arms strong and powerful with shoulders back and collarbones wide. Keep the abdominals drawn in.

*Traditionally this exercise is performed to the instruction of 'inhale for five beats and exhale for five beats until you reach 100'.

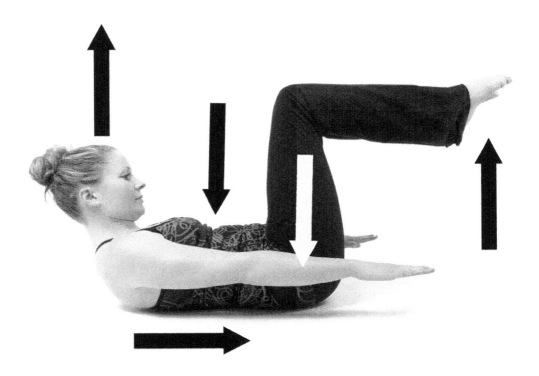

One Hundred 2
(Advanced)

AIM: To strengthen the abdominals and increase the heart rate.

Opposition:

↑ UP: Create a sense of length out through the legs and lengthen out through the top of the head.

↓ DOWN: Maintain a positive connection between the ribcage and the floor. Allow the pelvis to drop heavily into the floor, *in opposition* to the lift of the upper body and the length of the legs.

OTHER (energy): Send the arms away from you alongside the body with the shoulders back and the fingers long and strong.

Directions:

From **One Hundred 1**, stretch the legs out to a 70 degree angle (or lower if you are stronger) and position them either in parallel (together) or turned out from the feet and hips. **Inhale** and **exhale** fully for a count of 10 as you pump the arms up and down vigorously, from in line with the body to slightly above and back again.*

Other considerations:

Keep the arms strong and powerful with shoulders back and collarbones wide. Keep the abdominals drawn in. Stretch through the knees and squeeze the inner thighs together.

Traditionally this exercise is performed to the instruction of, 'inhale for five beats and exhale for five beats until you reach 100'.

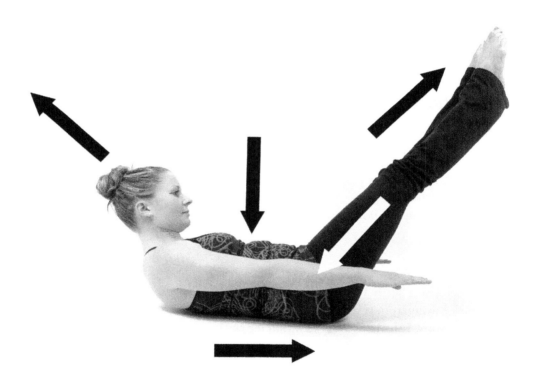

Single Leg Stretch 1

AIM: To strengthen the abdominals and improve quadriceps and hip flexor strength/control.

Opposition:

↑ UP: Create a sense of lightness out of the crown of the head. Lengthen one leg away from you.

↓ DOWN: Maintain a positive connection between the ribcage and the floor. Allow the pelvis to drop heavily into the floor, *in opposition* to the lift of the upper body and the length of the leg.

Directions:

From **Curl Up 3 with Double Knee Fold, inhale** to prepare. As you **exhale**, send one leg away from you to a 45 degree angle. Allow the other leg to draw toward you very slightly. **Inhale** as you draw that leg back in, *as if you had springs connected to your toes,* and **exhale** to stretch the other leg away.

Other considerations:

Keep the heels of both feet in a horizontal line with each other as you stretch one away. Keep the abdominals drawn in throughout. Keep the head heavy in the hands.

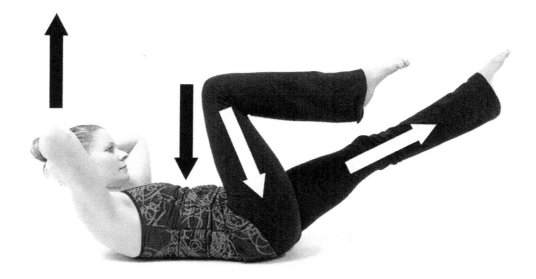

Single Leg Stretch 2

AIM: To strengthen the abdominals and improve quadriceps and hip flexor strength/ control.

Opposition:

↑ **UP:**   Create a sense of lightness out of the crown of the head. Lengthen one leg away from you.

↓ **DOWN:**   Maintain a positive connection between the ribcage and the floor. Allow the pelvis to drop heavily into the floor, *in opposition* to the lift of the upper body and the length of the leg.

Directions:

From **Single Leg Stretch 1**, take the same side hand of the bent knee to the ankle. Take the opposite (free) hand to the knee. **Inhale** to prepare; as you **exhale**, send the free leg away from you to a 45 degree angle. Gently draw the other leg toward you. **Inhale** as you pull the straight leg back in, *as if you had springs connected to your toes,* and **exhale** to change arms and stretch the other leg away.

Other considerations:

Keep the heels of both feet in a horizontal line with each other as you stretch one away. Keep the abdominals drawn in throughout. Keep the head heavy in the hands. Try to avoid compressing the hip and knee joints with your hands.

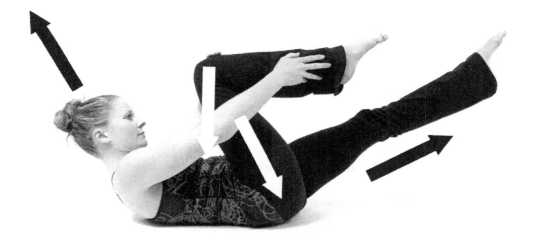

Double Leg Stretch 1

AIM: To strengthen the abdominals and improve quadriceps and hip flexor strength/control.

Opposition:

↑ UP: Create a sense of length through the legs and lengthen out through the top of the head.

↓ DOWN: Maintain a positive connection between the ribcage and the floor. Allow the pelvis to drop heavily into the floor, *in opposition* to the lift of the upper body and the length through the legs.

Directions:

From **One Hundred 1**, **exhale** to prepare. **Inhale** as you stretch the legs out to a 70 degree angle (or lower if you are stronger) and position them either in parallel (together) or turned out from the feet and hips. Lift the arms up at the same time so that they are parallel to the legs.* As you **exhale**, draw the legs back in, *as if you had springs connected to your toes,* and lower the arms to the starting position.

Other considerations:

Stretch the arms toward your toes as you lift them up, keeping the shoulders back and the collarbones wide.

You can keep the hands behind the head if you are experiencing neck strain as if you were in **Curl Up.**

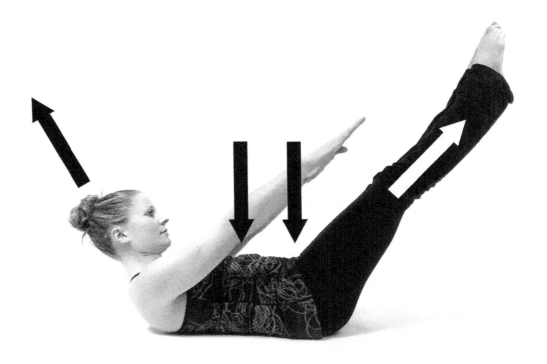

Double Leg Stretch 2
(Advanced)

AIM: To strengthen the abdominals and improve quadriceps and hip flexor strength/control. To improve shoulder stability and scapulohumeral rhythm.*

Opposition:

↑ UP: Create a sense of length through the legs and lengthen out through the top of the head and arms.

↓ DOWN: Maintain a positive connection between the ribcage and the floor. Allow the pelvis to drop heavily into the floor, *in opposition* to the lift of the upper body and the length through the legs.

Directions:

From **double leg stretch 1**, **inhale** to take the arms parallel to your straight legs. **Exhale** and stretch the arms over your head, sweeping them out to the sides and simultaneously drawing the legs back in toward your starting position, *as if your toes were connected to springs.*

Other considerations:

Make sure that your arm circle stays within your peripheral vision. Avoid falling backward out of your curl up as the weight of your arms moves over your head. Keep the abdominals drawn in throughout.

*Scapulohumeral rhythm is the biomechanically efficient relationship between the shoulder blade (scapula), humerus (upper arm bone) and clavicles (collarbones).

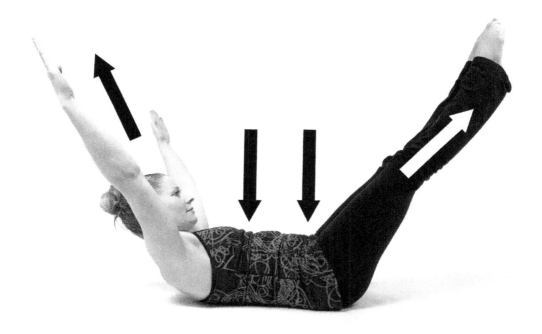

Sitting
(Preparation)

AIM: To lengthen the spinal column.

Opposition:

↑ UP: Create a sense of length through the crown of the head.

↓ DOWN: Feel the weight of your sitting bones increasing as you lengthen away *in opposition*.

Directions:

Sit tall with your knees bent and your feet flat on the floor. **Inhale** and **exhale** in a steady and controlled manner as you lengthen the spine.

Other considerations:

Avoid gripping in the hips and thighs (quadriceps). Keep the shoulders back and the collarbones wide.

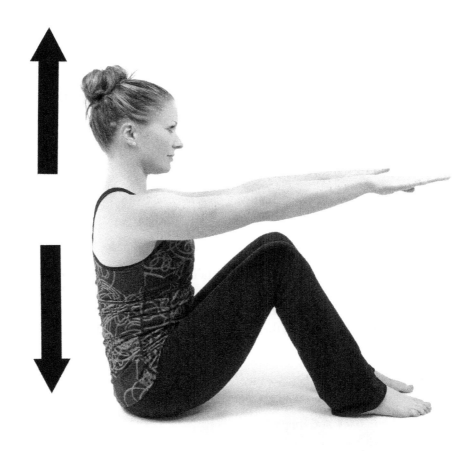

Half Roll Back ('C' Curve)

AIM: To strengthen the lower abdominals and stretch the lumbar (lower) spine.

Opposition:

↑ UP: Create a sense of length through the arms.

↓ DOWN: Draw the abdominals in, away (*in opposition*) from the fingertips.

Directions:

From your **Sitting** position, **inhale** and lengthen up. As you **exhale**, squeeze your buttocks and roll them backward underneath you.* Once you are behind your sitting bones, you can relax the squeeze. **Inhale** to tilt your curved spine forward, keeping the lower back long, then re-stack the spinal column as you **exhale**.

Other considerations:

Avoid gripping in the hips and thighs (quadriceps). Keep the feet flat on the floor. Keep the shoulders back and the collarbones wide.

Try not to think about 'traveling' backward. Focus on the tilt of the pelvis and the muscle activity that is both simultaneously created by and needed for the action.

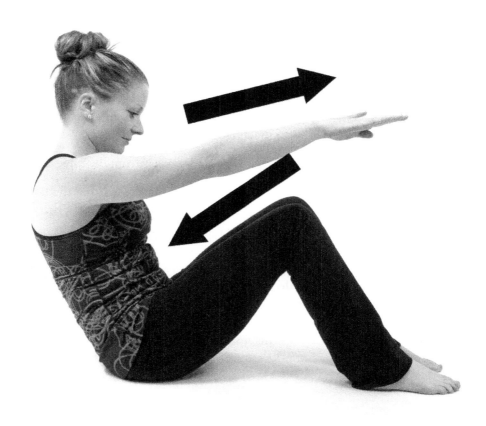

The Roll Back 1*

AIM: To strengthen the lower abdominals and stretch the lumbar (lower) spine. To mobilize the whole spinal column.

Opposition:

↑ UP:
1. Create a sense of length through the arms.
2. Stretch the arms over your head, keeping them in your peripheral vision, *in opposition* to the length in your thigh bones.

↓ DOWN:
1. Draw the abdominals in, away (*in opposition*) from the fingertips.
2. Maintain a strong connection between the ribcage and the floor. Keep the pelvis heavy.

Directions:

From your **Sitting** position, **inhale** and lengthen up. As you **exhale**, squeeze your buttocks and roll them backward underneath you. Keep rolling the spine down to the floor bone by bone until your head is in contact with the floor and the arms are over your head. **Inhale** to lift the arms up and start to roll the spine back up until you can re-stack the spinal column as you **exhale**.

Other considerations:

Avoid gripping in the hips and thighs (quadriceps). Keep the feet flat on the floor. Keep the shoulders back and the collarbones wide.

*In many ways this bent knees version of the roll back is actually harder than performing it with straight legs (as in **The Roll Back 2**) because the shorter lever does not assist with counterbalancing the action. If this is the case, start with **The Roll Back 2**.

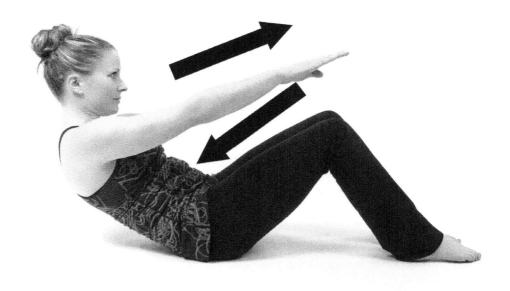

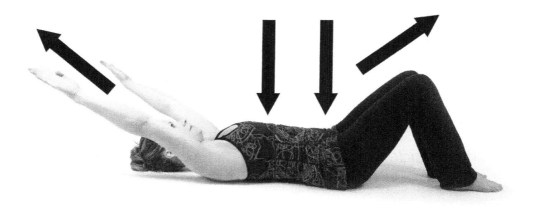

The Roll Back 2

AIM: To strengthen the lower abdominals and stretch the lumbar (lower) spine. To mobilize the whole spinal column.

Opposition:

↑ UP: 1. Create a sense of length through the arms throughout the movement.

2. Stretch the crown of the head away from the legs and feet.

3. Lengthen out through the arms.

↓ DOWN: 1, 2 & 3. Draw the ribcage down and in toward the spine, and draw the abdominals in, away (*in opposition*) from the fingertips as you roll up and forward.

OTHER (energy): When lying out flat in the spine, lengthen the arms away *in opposition* to the length along the thighs (quadriceps). Keep the legs stretching away.

Directions:

From lying out flat, with the arms over your head in your peripheral vision, **inhale** and start to lift the arms and follow with the upper body. As you **exhale**, continue to roll all the way up into a forward **Spine Stretch**.

Other considerations:

Keep the legs straight and the feet in turnout (heels together, the outside edges of your feet directed away from each other). Try to limit the amount that your legs slide forward when you roll up.

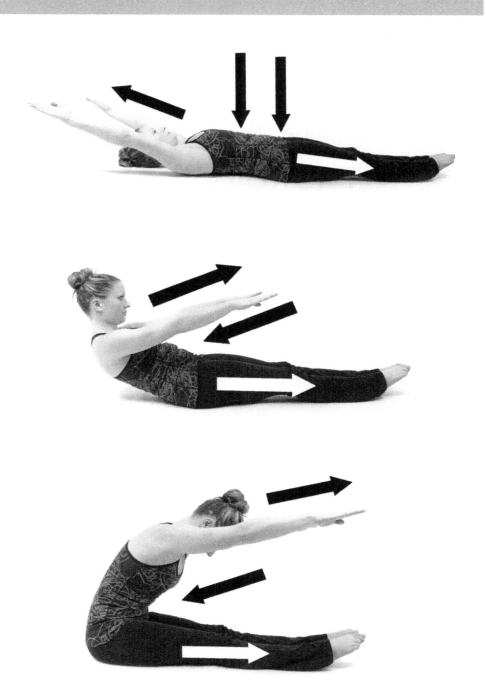

The Hip Lift /
The Roll Over 1

AIM: To strengthen the lower abdominals and stretch the lumbar (lower) spine.

Opposition:

↑ UP: Create a sense of length through the legs.

↓ DOWN: Draw the ribcage down and in toward the floor, and create a sense of heaviness in the pelvis.

Directions:

With the thigh bones vertical and the lower part of the legs extended to your most comfortable position, **inhale** and press the backs of your arms (triceps) into the floor. With control, **exhale** and aim to squeeze your hips up off the floor. Carefully lower back down as you **inhale**.

Other considerations:

Try to focus on control in the lift rather than using momentum. Keep the shoulders back and the collarbones wide.

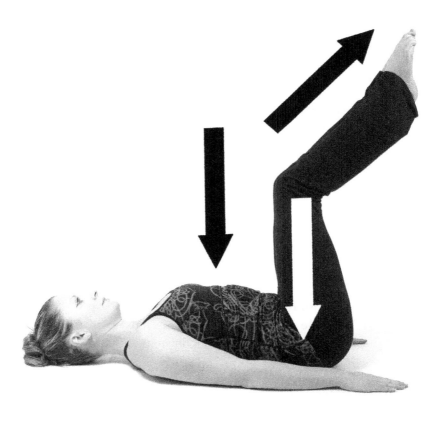

The Roll Over 2
(Advanced)

AIM: To strengthen the lower abdominals and stretch the lumbar (lower) spine. To mobilize the whole spinal column.

Opposition:

↑ **UP:**   Create a sense of length through the spine and legs.

↓ **DOWN:**   Press your upper arms (triceps) into the floor and create a sense of heaviness through the upper ribcage and the back of the shoulders.

Directions:

With the legs straight, **inhale** and press the backs of your arms (triceps) into the floor. With control, **exhale** and aim to squeeze your hips up off the floor and send the legs over your head.* Carefully lower back down as you **inhale**.

Other considerations:

Try to focus on control in the lift rather than using momentum. Keep the shoulders back and the collarbones wide.

Do not let the legs fall lower than the horizontal and avoid putting pressure on your neck.

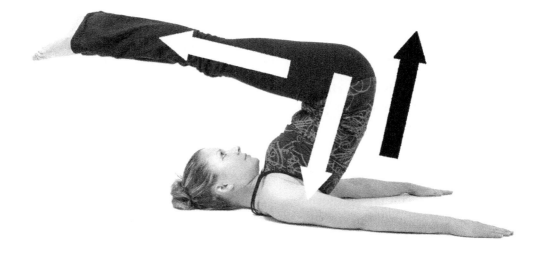

Upper Back Extension 1

AIM: To mobilize and strengthen the upper spine and associated muscles.

Opposition:

↑ UP: 1. Create a sense of length out through the crown of the head.

↓ DOWN: 1 & 2. Allow the chest to sink heavily into the floor and aim to balance the bones of the pelvis evenly and heavily (without squeezing the buttocks).

Directions:

Position the legs with the toes together and heels apart. Relax the buttocks. Place your fingertips together and rest your forehead on them. **Inhale** to prepare; as you **exhale** allow the chest to become heavier and pull the back of your head toward the ceiling to create lift. Keep your eyeline down. **Inhale** to lower back down.

Other considerations:

Avoid gripping in your legs and buttocks as you lift. Keep the shoulders relaxed and the arms light. Maintain length in the back of the neck.

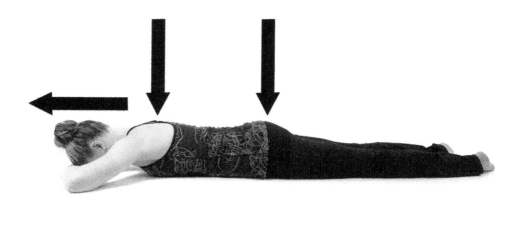

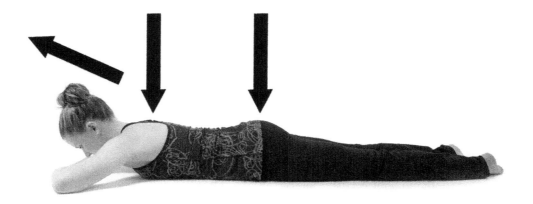

Upper Back Extension 2

AIM: To mobilize and strengthen the upper spine and associated muscles.

Opposition:

↑ UP: Create a sense of length out through the crown of the head.

↓ DOWN: Allow the chest to sink heavily into the floor and aim to balance the bones of the pelvis evenly and heavily (without squeezing the buttocks).

Directions:

Position the legs shoulder distance apart with feet slightly turned out. Relax the buttocks. Place your arms by the sides of your head with the elbows at ribcage level and the fingertips at head level. The lower arms should be in line with your body. **Inhale** to prepare; as you **exhale** allow the chest to become heavier and pull the back of your head toward the ceiling to create lift.* Keep your eyeline down. **Inhale** to lower back down.

Other considerations:

Avoid gripping in your legs and buttocks as you lift. Keep the shoulders relaxed and the arms light. Maintain length in the back of the neck.

*You will naturally achieve more height than in **Upper Back Extension 1**.

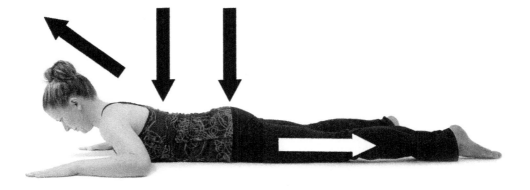

Cobra /
Upper Back Extension 3

AIM: To mobilize and strengthen the upper spine and associated muscles. To strengthen the buttocks.

Opposition:

↑ UP: Create a sense of length out through the crown of the head.

↓ DOWN: Press the pelvis into the floor, squeezing the buttocks.

Other (energy): Create a strong connection between the hands and the floor and lengthen the legs away from you.

Directions:

From the **exhaled** lift of **Upper Back Extension 2**, **inhale** and squeeze the buttocks and press with the arms to continue rolling the spine up into a more lifted position. **Exhale** to lower back down.

Other considerations:

It is not necessary to straighten your arms – work within your most comfortable range. Keep the shoulders down and the neck long. Your eyeline will travel along the floor and up the wall, so that you end up looking directly forward, avoiding over-arching/hyper-extending your neck.

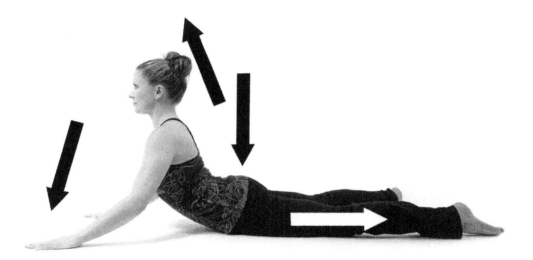

Swan Dive 1 /
Upper Back Extension 4
(Advanced)

AIM: To mobilize and strengthen the upper spine and associated muscles. To strengthen the buttocks. To lengthen the hip flexors.

Opposition:

↑ UP: Create a sense of length out through the crown of the head. Maintain lightness in the back of the legs.

↓ DOWN: Press the pelvis into the floor, squeezing the buttocks.

Other (energy): Create a sense of length out of the legs (stretch the knees).

Directions:

From the **inhaled** lift of **Cobra/Upper Back Extension 3**, **exhale** and lower the body down the forearms, keep the buttocks active and allow the legs to lift up behind you. **Inhale** to return to **Cobra**, with the legs down and the body lifted.

Other considerations:

Keep the shoulders down and the neck long. Avoid over-arching/hyper-extending your neck.

Keep the knees straight.

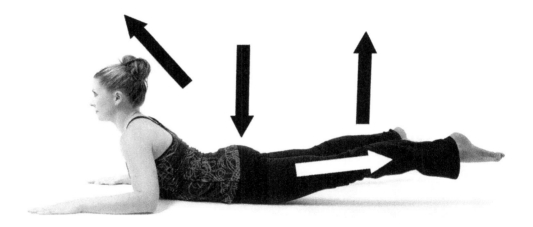

Swan Dive 2
(Advanced)

AIM: To mobilize and strengthen the upper spine and associated muscles. To strengthen the buttocks. To lengthen the hip flexors.

Opposition:

↑ UP: Create a sense of length out through the crown of the head. Maintain lightness in the back of the legs.

↓ DOWN: Press the pelvis into the floor, squeezing the buttocks.

Other (energy): Create a sense of length out of the legs (stretch the knees).

Directions:

From the **inhaled** lift of **Cobra/Upper Back Extension 3**, **exhale** and throw your arms forward. You will rock forward on your pelvis, the legs lifting up behind you. DO NOT LOOK DOWN. As you **inhale** and rock backward, place your hands back down on the floor to catch yourself in **Cobra**.

Other considerations:

Keep the shoulders down and the neck long. Avoid over-arching/hyper-extending your neck.

Keep the knees straight.

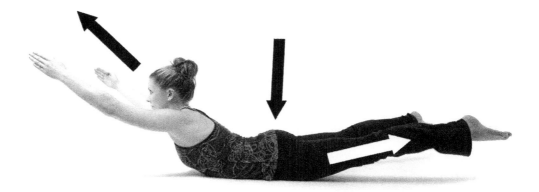

Oyster /
Side Lying Legs 1

AIM: To strengthen the stabilizing muscles of the pelvis.

Opposition:

↑ UP: Create a sense of length out through the crown of the head and out through the top thigh bone.

↓ DOWN: Press the hand into the floor.

Directions:

Lie on your side and bend your knees. Place your feet and lower arm in line with your spine. Place the other arm in front of you for support. Lift up the feet so that they are in line with the center of your buttocks. **Inhale** to prepare; as you **exhale**, lift up the top leg, keeping the pelvis level. **Inhale** to lower.

Other considerations:

Keep the shoulders down and the neck long. Keep the ribcage drawn in toward the spine and the waistline long.

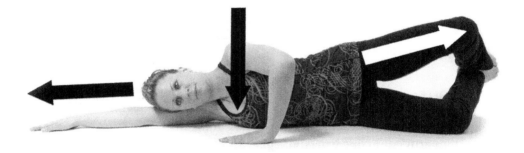

Side Lying Legs 2

AIM: To strengthen the stabilizing muscles of the pelvis.

Opposition:

↑ UP: 1. Create a sense of length out through the top leg/heel.

↓ DOWN: 1 & 2. Press the hand into the floor.

Other (energy): Stretch out through the crown of the head *in opposition* to the leg.

Directions:

Lie on your side and bend your bottom knee to 90 degrees in front of you. Stretch your bottom arm out in line with your spine and stretch the top leg out in line with the top of your hip. Flex the foot. **Inhale** to prepare; as you **exhale**, send your top leg forward, keeping the pelvis still. **Inhale** and point your toes to return, squeezing the buttocks to take the legs slightly behind you, opening up the hip.

Other considerations:

Keep the shoulders down and the neck long. Keep the ribcage drawn in toward the spine and the waistline long.

Keep the knee straight.

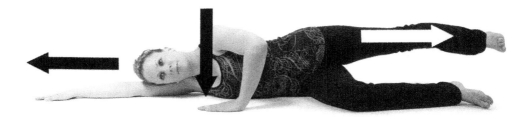

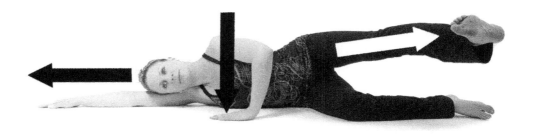

Side Lying Legs 3

AIM: To strengthen the stabilizing muscles of the pelvis.

Opposition:

↑ UP: 1 & 2. Create a sense of length out through the top leg/toes.

↓ DOWN: 1 & 2. Press the hand into the floor.

Other (energy): Stretch out through the crown of the head and arm *in opposition* to the stationary leg.

Directions:

Lie on your side and stretch your bottom leg out to 45 degrees. Stretch your bottom arm out in line with your spine and stretch the top leg out in line with the top of your hip. Point the foot and turn it out. **Inhale** to prepare; as you **exhale**, send your top leg forward, keeping the pelvis still. **Inhale** and flex your foot to return, squeezing the buttocks to take the legs slightly behind you, opening up the hip.

Other considerations:

Keep the shoulders down and the neck long. Keep the ribcage drawn in toward the spine and the waistline long.

Keep the knee straight.

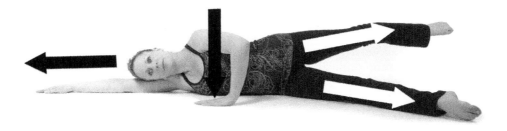

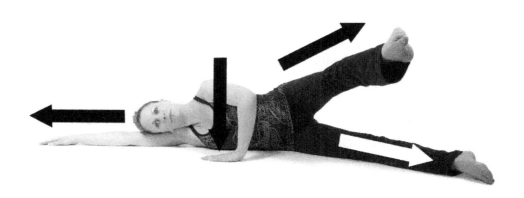

Side Lying Legs 4
(Advanced)

AIM: To strengthen the stabilizing muscles of the pelvis.

Opposition:

↑ UP: Create a sense of length out through the crown of the head and out through both legs.

↓ DOWN: Press the hand into the floor.

Directions:

Lie on your side and straighten both legs to a 45 degree angle in front of you. Lift up your upper body and place your hand behind your head. Use your free hand for support in front of you. **Inhale** to prepare; as you **exhale**, kick the top leg up and out with pointed toes, keeping the pelvis still and the leg directly over the bottom one.* **Inhale** to lower with control, *as if you are squeezing through treacle.*

Other considerations:

Keep the shoulders down and the neck long. Keep the ribcage drawn in toward the spine and the waistline long (optional: flex the foot as you lower).

The more you stretch the leg out, the lower the kick and the longer the waistline.

Keep the knees straight.

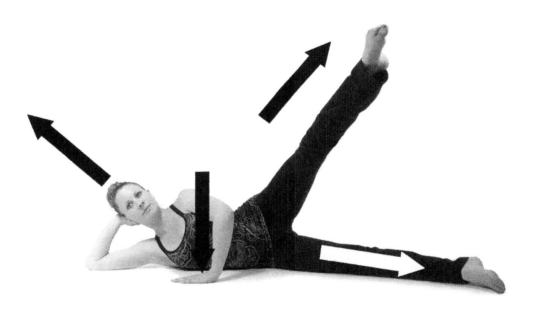

Side Lying Legs 5

(Advanced)

AIM: To strengthen the stabilizing muscles of the pelvis.

Opposition:

↑ UP:　　Create a sense of length out through the crown of the head and out through the top leg.

↓ DOWN:　Draw the ribcage in toward the spine and stretch the bottom leg out along the floor.

Directions:

Lie on your side and straighten both legs to a 45 degree angle in front of you. Lift up your upper body and place both your hands behind your head. Keep your ribcage drawn in. **Inhale** to prepare; as you **exhale**, kick the top leg up and out with pointed toes, keeping the pelvis still and the leg directly over the bottom one.* **Inhale** to lower with control, *as if you are squeezing through treacle.*

Other considerations:

Keep the shoulders down and the neck long. Use your hands to create more length in the neck. Keep the ribcage drawn in toward the spine and the waistline long (optional: flex the foot as you lower).

The more you stretch the leg out, the lower the kick and the longer the waistline.

Keep the knees straight.

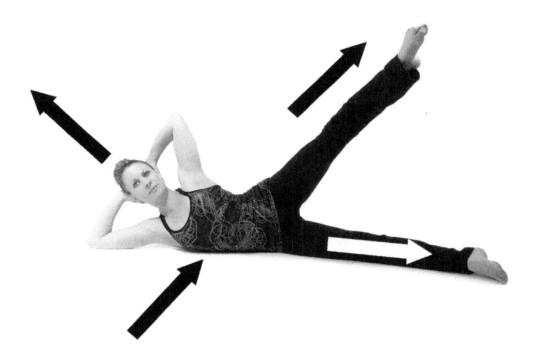

Mermaid 1

AIM: To stretch the obliques (sides).

Opposition:

↑ UP: 1 & 2. Create a sense of length out through the crown of the head and out through the arm.

↓ DOWN: 1 & 2. Allow the pelvis to drop heavily into the floor.

Directions:

Position your legs with knees bent and the feet pointing in the same direction. You may separate the legs if more comfortable. Hold on to your ankles with one hand and pull yourself into a tall sitting position. Raise the arm up so that it is softly straight and in front of your face. **Inhale** and lengthen, as you **exhale** gently bend toward your legs, keeping a sense of space through the shortening waistline. **Inhale** and lengthen back up.

Other considerations:

Keep the shoulders down and the neck long. Keep the ribcage and abdominals drawn in toward the spine.

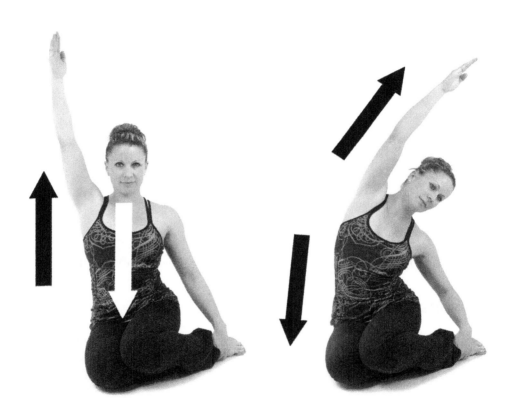

Mermaid 2 /
Side Hip Lift

AIM: To stretch and strengthen the obliques (sides).

Opposition:

↑ UP: Send the ribcage toward the ceiling.

↓ DOWN: Maintain a positive connection with the knees.

Other (energy): Create a sense of length through the crown of the head and arm.

Directions:

From **Mermaid 1, inhale** and send your body in the other direction. Position your forearm on the floor and **exhale** to lift your body up, keeping the knees together. **Inhale** to transition smoothly back to **Mermaid 1**. **Exhale** and stretch.

Other considerations:

Keep the shoulders down and the neck long. Keep the ribcage and abdominals drawn in toward the spine.

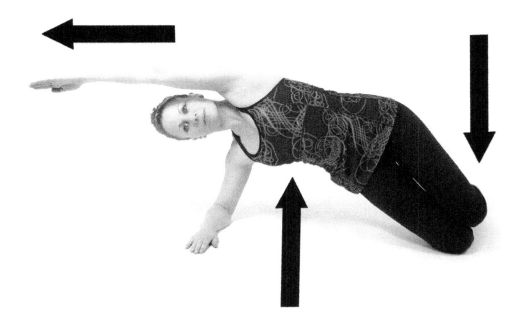

Side Twist 1 / Mermaid 3
(Advanced)

AIM: To stretch and strengthen the obliques (sides).

Opposition:

↑ UP: 1. Create a sense of length out through the crown of the head.

2. Lift through the ribcage.

↓ DOWN: 1. Allow the pelvis to drop heavily into the floor.

2. Maintain a strong connection through the hands and feet.

Other (energy):

1. Stretch the arm away from you as it presses the top knee back.

2. Stretch the arm away from you over your head.

Directions:

Position your legs with your bottom knee bent, foot in line with the buttocks. Place your top foot flat on the floor in front of your ankle. Use your arm to push the top knee back and sit heavily into the pelvis. Position the other hand firmly on the floor, a little distance away from you. **Inhale** to lengthen the spine. **Exhale** and press your hand and top foot into the floor to lift the whole body up into a side bend. Sweep your free arm over your head. **Inhale** to return to the starting position.

Other considerations:

Keep the shoulders down and the neck long. Keep the ribcage and abdominals drawn in toward the spine.

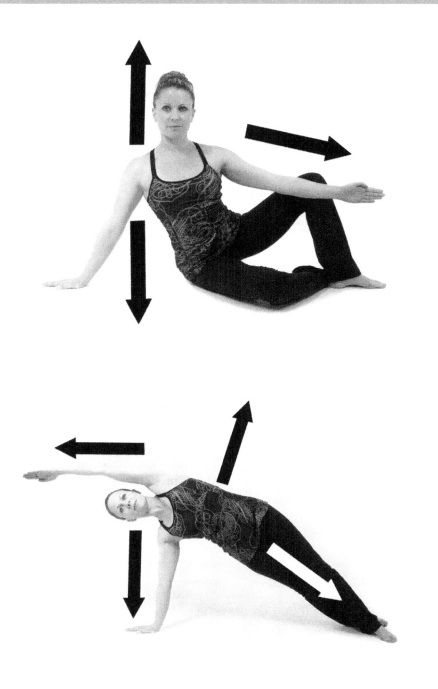

Side Twist 2 / Mermaid 4

(Advanced)

AIM: To stretch and strengthen the obliques (sides).

Opposition:

↑ UP: 1. Create a sense of lift at the ribcage.

2. Create a sense of lift through the hips.

↓ DOWN: 1 & 2. Maintain a strong connection through the hand and feet

Other (energy): Stretch the arm over your head in opposition to the legs. Stretch the arm through underneath your body.

Directions:

From **Side Twist 1/ Mermaid 3**, **inhale** to prepare; as you **exhale**, rotate the upper body, lifting your hips up and dropping the upper body down so that you can stretch your free arm underneath the body. **Inhale** to roll back up to the side stretch, **exhale** to return to the **Side Twist/Mermaid 3** sitting position.

Other considerations:

Keep the shoulders down and the neck long. Keep the ribcage and abdominals drawn in toward the spine.

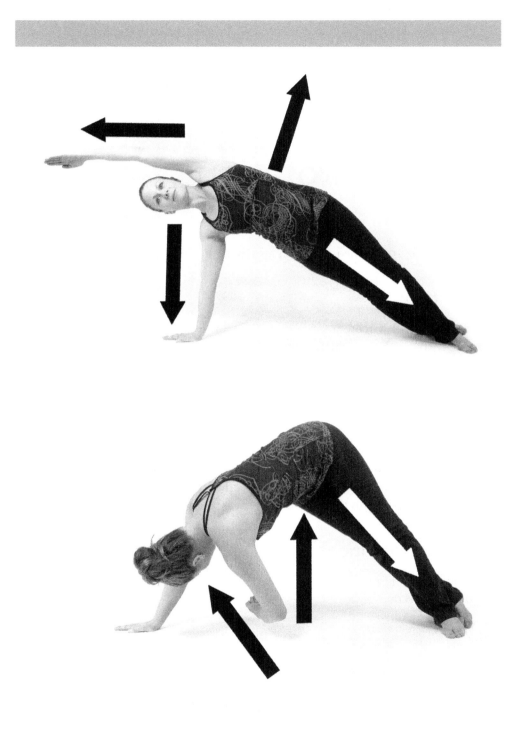

Rotation 1

AIM: To mobilize the spine in rotation and work the obliques.

Opposition:

↑ UP: 1 & 2. Create a sense of lightness through the back of the neck and through the spine.

↓ DOWN: 1 & 2. Maintain a sense of heaviness through the pelvis.

Directions:

Sit with the soles of your feet together and the knees dropped out to the sides.* Place your hands behind your head and gently lift the head away from the shoulders. **Exhale** to prepare; as you **inhale**, twist the body in one direction, keeping the pelvis level. **Exhale** to return to the center and repeat on the other side.

Other considerations:

Keep the shoulders down and the neck long. Keep the ribcage and abdominals drawn in toward the spine.

You may feel more comfortable sitting on a block or a pillow.

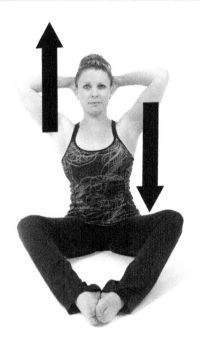

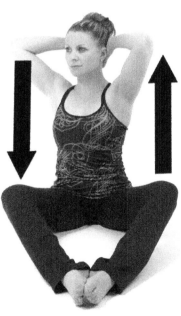

Rotation 2

AIM: To mobilize the spine in rotation and work the obliques.

Opposition:

↑ UP: Create a sense of lightness through the back of the neck and through the spine.

↓ DOWN: Maintain a sense of heaviness through the pelvis.

Other (energy): Stretch the arms away from each other in opposite directions.

Directions:

Sit with your legs out straight in front of you, feet flexed.* Stretch your arms out to the sides, level with and just in front of your collarbones. **Exhale** to prepare; as you **inhale**, twist the body in one direction, keeping the pelvis level and the arms slightly in front of your collarbones. **Exhale** to return to the center and repeat on the other side.

Other considerations:

Keep the shoulders down and the neck long. Keep the ribcage and abdominals drawn in toward the spine.

You may feel more comfortable sitting on a block or a pillow.

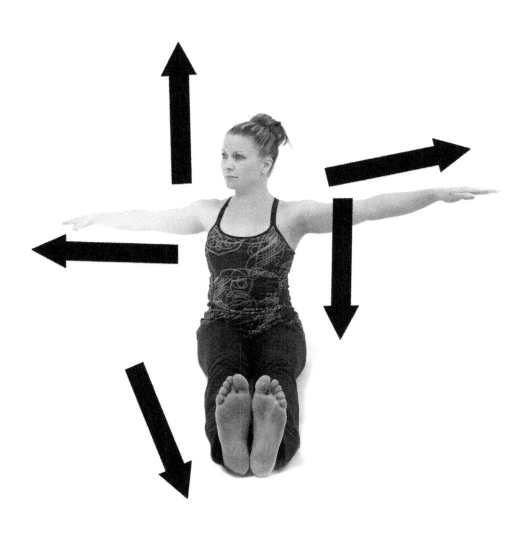

The Saw / Rotation 3
(Advanced)

AIM: To mobilize the spine in rotation and work the obliques.

Opposition:

↑ UP: Create a sense of lightness through the back of the neck and through the spine.

        1. Stretch the back arm up and away from the front arm.

↓ DOWN: 1 & 2. Maintain a sense of heaviness through the pelvis.

        2. Stretch the front arm away toward the little toe and away from the back arm *in opposition*.

Other (energy): Stretch the arms and legs away from each other *in opposition*.

Directions:

Sit with your legs stretched out to the sides, as wide as possible, feet flexed.* Stretch your arms out to the sides, level with and just in front of your collarbones. **Exhale** to prepare; as you **inhale**, twist the body in one direction, keeping the pelvis level and the arms slightly in front of your collarbones. **Exhale** and stretch forward, reaching your arm toward the opposite foot. Direct your little finger toward your little toe. Reach the free arm behind, up and away from the other arm.

Other considerations:

Keep the shoulders down and the neck long. Keep the ribcage and abdominals drawn in toward the spine.

You may feel more comfortable sitting on a block or a pillow.

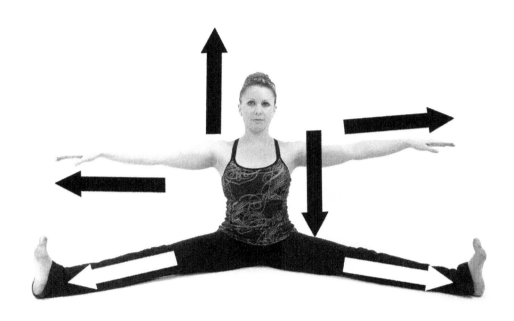

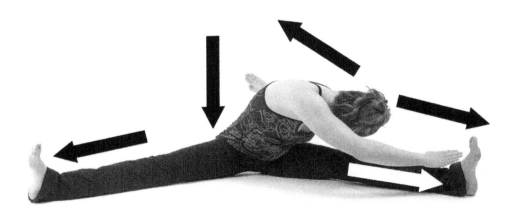

Cat

AIM: To mobilize the spine and strengthen the lower abdominals.

Opposition:

↑ UP: 1 & 2. Create a sense of lift through the bottom of the ribcage and lower abdominals.

↓ DOWN: 1 & 2. Maintain a strong connection through the whole of the hand.

2. Drop the head and tailbone down to the floor.

Other (energy): Stretch the crown of the head and the tailbone away from each other.

Directions:

Position your body in a four-point kneeling position, with the hands* directly underneath the shoulders and the knees directly underneath the hips. Lengthen the spine. **Inhale**; then as you **exhale**, tuck the buttocks under, sending your spine to the ceiling and your head and tailbone to the floor. DO NOT SQUEEZE YOUR BUTTOCKS AND LEGS. Hold the position and take a full **inhale** to the back and sides of your ribcage. **Exhale** to lengthen out of the position.

Other considerations:

Keep the shoulders down and the neck long. Keep the ribcage and abdominals drawn in toward the spine.

If this makes your wrists uncomfortable, try balancing on fists.

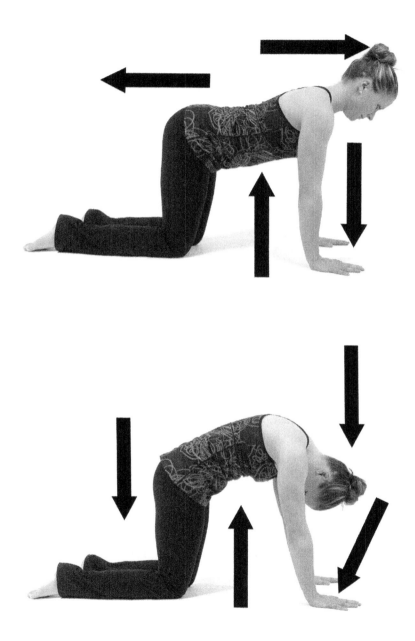

Table Top 1

AIM: To strengthen the obliques and improve balance.

Opposition:

↑ UP: Create a sense of length through the back of the neck and out through the crown of the head. Maintain a sense of lift through the bottom of the ribcage.

↓ DOWN: Maintain a strong connection between ONE hand and the floor. Lengthen out through the moving leg.

Directions:

Position your body in a four-point kneeling position, with the hands* directly underneath the shoulders and the knees directly underneath the hips. Lengthen the spine. **Inhale** to prepare; then as you **exhale**, transfer your body weight on to one supporting hand and the opposite knee. When the leg on the same side as the supporting hand starts to feel light, slide the leg away; keep it on the floor and avoid rocking the body to one side. **Inhale** and lengthen through the spine and leg. As you **exhale**, pull the leg back in *as if your toes were attached to springs.*

Other considerations:

Keep the shoulders down and the neck long. Keep the ribcage and abdominals drawn in toward the spine.

If this makes your wrists uncomfortable, try balancing on fists.

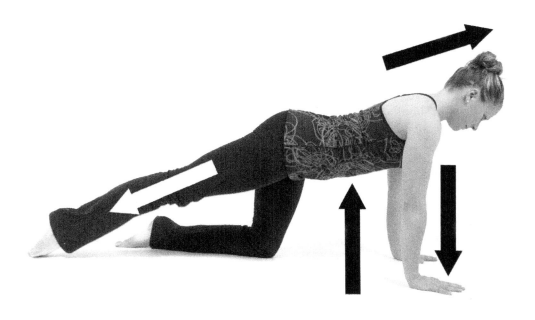

Superman / Table Top 2

AIM: To strengthen the obliques and improve balance.

Opposition:

↑ UP: Create a sense of length through the back of the neck and out through the crown of the head. Maintain a sense of lift through the bottom of the ribcage.

↓ DOWN: Maintain a strong connection between ONE hand, ONE knee and the floor. Lengthen out through the moving leg.

Directions:

Position your body in a four-point kneeling position, with the hands* directly underneath the shoulders and the knees directly underneath the hips. Lengthen the spine. **Inhale** to prepare; then as you **exhale**, transfer your body weight on to one supporting hand and the opposite knee. The other hand and knee will start to feel light. Slide the light leg and opposite arm away. Lift the arm and leg away from the floor and avoid rocking the body to one side. **Inhale** and lengthen through the spine and stretched arm and leg. As you **exhale**, pull the arm and leg back in *as if your toes and fingers were attached to springs*.

Other considerations:

Keep the shoulders down and the neck long. Keep the ribcage and abdominals drawn in toward the spine.

If this makes your wrists uncomfortable, try balancing on fists.

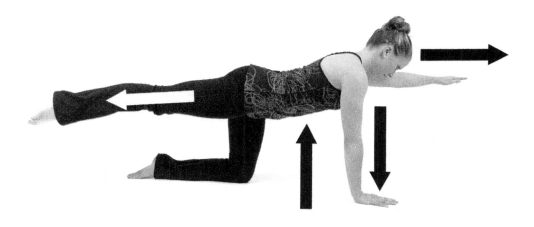

Leg Pull Front 1

AIM: To strengthen the abdominals and arms.

Opposition:

↑ UP: 1 & 2. Maintain a sense of lift through the bottom of the ribcage.

↓ DOWN: 1 & 2. Maintain a strong connection between the hands and the floor.

Other (energy):

1. Maintain a sense of length through the spine and out through the crown of the head. Lengthen the legs away *in opposition*.

2. When pulling one leg in, drive through the middle of the thigh rather than the knee.

Directions:

From **Superman/Table Top 2***, slide the other leg out so that you end up in a 'plank position'. **Inhale** to lengthen through the body. As you **exhale**, pull one leg in underneath the body, keeping the top of the foot on the floor. **Inhale** to return the leg and change sides.

Other considerations:

Keep the shoulders down and the neck long. Keep the ribcage and abdominals drawn in toward the spine.

*If this makes your wrists uncomfortable, try balancing on fists.

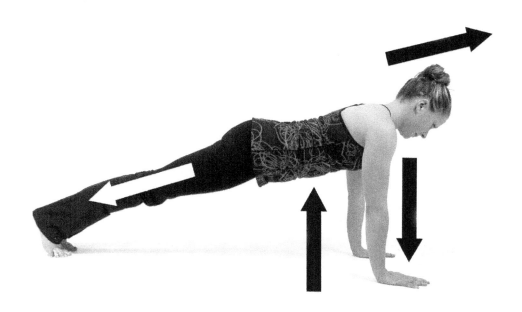

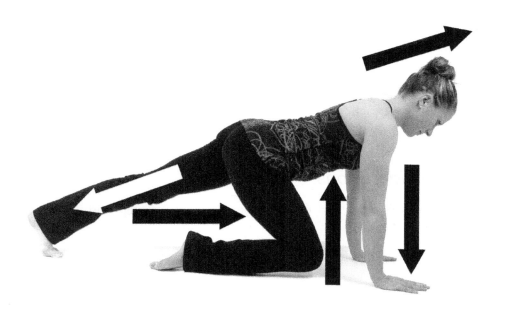

Leg Pull Front 2
(Advanced)

AIM: To strengthen the abdominals, arms and buttocks.

Opposition:

↑ UP: 1 & 2. Maintain a sense of lift through the bottom of the ribcage.

↓ DOWN: 1 & 2. Maintain a strong connection between the hands and the floor.

Other (energy): Maintain a sense of length through the spine and out through the crown of the head. Lengthen the legs away *in opposition*.

Directions:

From **Leg Pull 1*** starting position, **inhale** and lengthen through the whole body. As you **exhale**, push one heel toward the floor and lift the other leg up and away. Squeeze the buttock of the lifting leg and keep the knee straight. **Inhale** to return and then change sides.

Other considerations:

Keep the shoulders down and the neck long. Keep the ribcage and abdominals drawn in toward the spine.

*If this makes your wrists uncomfortable, try balancing on fists.

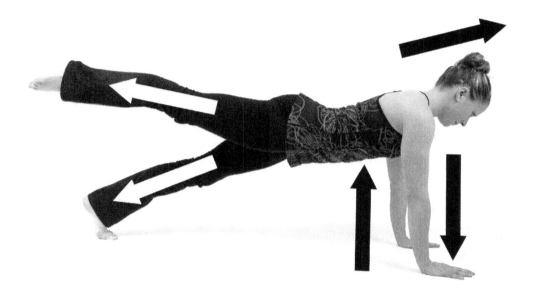

Leg Pull Back 1

AIM: To strengthen the triceps, hamstrings and buttocks.

Opposition:

↑ UP: 1 & 2. Maintain a sense of lift through the breastbone and out through the crown of the head.

2. Create a sense of lift from underneath the buttocks.

↓ DOWN: 1 & 2. Maintain a strong connection between the hands and the floor. Create a sense of heaviness through the pelvis.

Other (energy): Maintain a sense of length through the spine, through the back of the neck and out through the crown of the head. Lengthen the legs away *in opposition.*

Directions:

Sit with your legs out straight and arms behind you, hands facing the feet.* You should feel as if you are leaning slightly backward. **Inhale** and lengthen through the body; as you **exhale,** tuck the tailbone slightly under and then lift the hips up by squeezing the buttocks and lengthening through the legs. Push your body out of your shoulders. **Inhale** to lower back down.

Other considerations:

Avoid throwing the head backward, your eyeline should look 45 degrees away from you.

If this makes your wrists uncomfortable, try turning the hands out so that they are pointing away from your sides i.e. not pointing behind you.

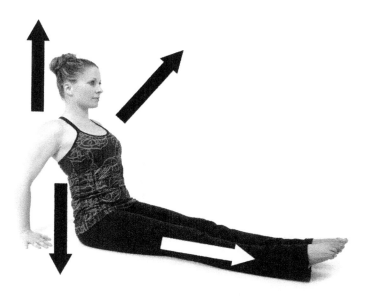

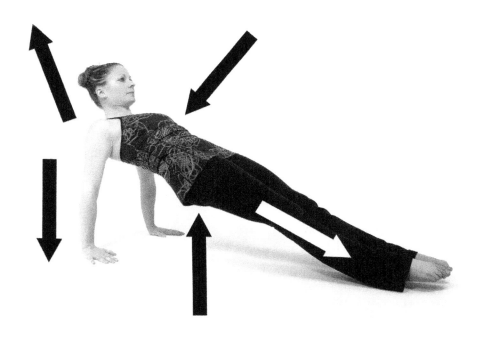

Leg Pull Back 2

AIM: To strengthen the triceps, hamstrings and buttocks.

Opposition:

↑ UP: 1 & 2. Maintain a sense of lift through the breastbone and out through the crown of the head.

        2. Create a sense of lift from underneath the buttocks.

↓ DOWN: 1 & 2. Maintain a strong connection between the hands and the floor.

Other (energy): Maintain a sense of length through the spine, through the back of the neck and out through the crown of the head. Lengthen the legs away *in opposition.*

Directions:

From **Leg Pull 1** *ending* position, **inhale** and lengthen through the whole body. As you **exhale**, bend one knee and slide the foot along the floor and in toward your buttocks. **Inhale** and slide the leg back to the start. **Exhale** to change sides.

Other considerations:

Avoid throwing the head backward, your eyeline should look 45 degrees away from you. Keep the pelvis level.

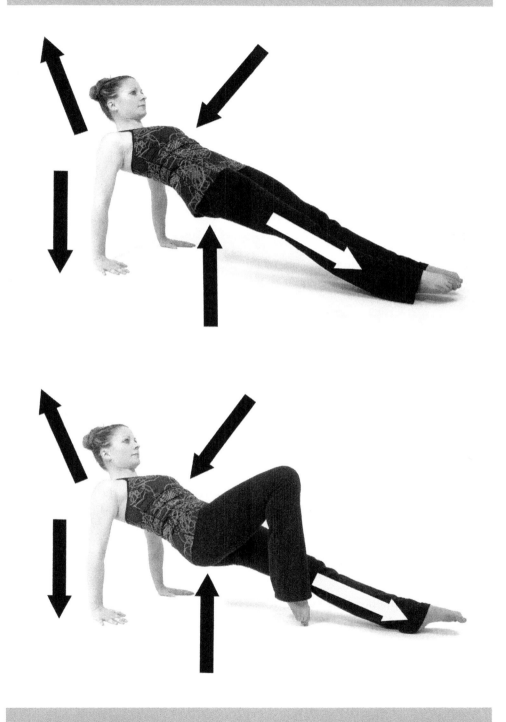

Leg Pull Back 3
(Advanced)

AIM: To strengthen the triceps, hamstrings, quadriceps and buttocks.

Opposition:

↑ UP: 1 & 2. Maintain a sense of lift through the breastbone and out through the crown of the head.

2. Create a sense of lift from underneath the buttocks.

2. Create a sense of length through the kicking leg.

↓ DOWN: 1 & 2. Maintain a strong connection between the hands and the floor.

Other (energy): Maintain a sense of length through the spine, through the back of the neck and out through the crown of the head. Lengthen the leg away *in opposition.*

Directions:

From **Leg Pull 1** *ending* position, **inhale** and lengthen through the whole body. As you **exhale**, kick one leg toward the ceiling.* **Inhale** to lower and then **exhale** to change sides.

Other considerations:

Avoid throwing the head backward, your eyeline should look 45 degrees away from you. Keep the pelvis level.

*Avoid dropping the hips as you kick.

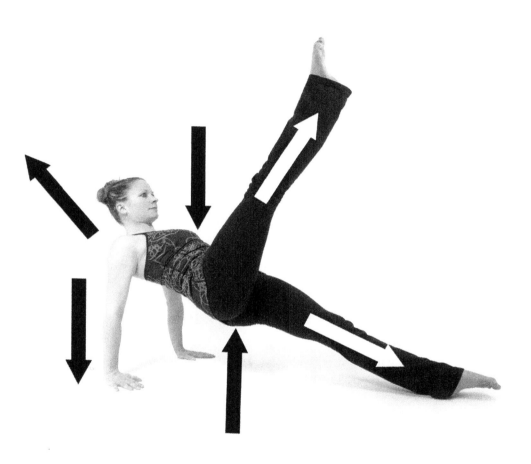

The Jack Knife
(Advanced)

AIM: To strengthen the buttocks and triceps. To mobilize the spine.

Opposition:

↑ UP: 1 & 2. Create a sense of length through the legs.

↓ DOWN: 1. Create a strong sense of connection through the ribcage and heaviness through the pelvis.

2. Maintain a strong connection between the backs of the arms and floor.

Directions:

Lie on your back with your legs vertical. **Inhale** and lengthen the spine; as you **exhale,** drive the legs straight up as vertically as you can. **Inhale** and lengthen through the body, and then **exhale** to slowly lower one bone at a time.

Other considerations:

Avoid balancing on your head and neck. Keep your lower arms and hands connected to the floor at all times.

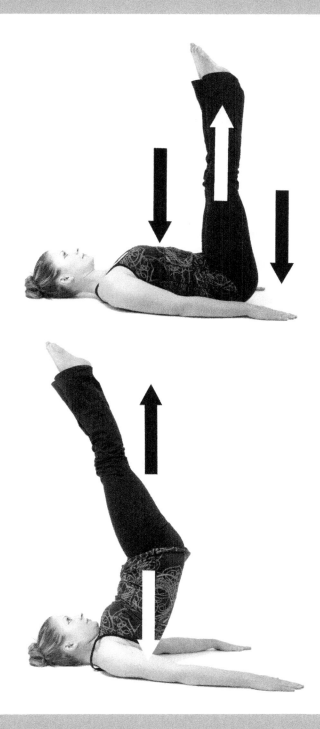

Scissors
(Advanced)

AIM: To lengthen the hip flexors, strengthen the buttocks and strengthen the abdominals.

Opposition:

↑ UP: 1 & 2. Maintain a sense of lift through the hips and length through the legs.

↓ DOWN: 1 & 2. Maintain a strong connection between the backs of the arms and the floor.

Directions:

From **The Jack Knife**, place your hands underneath your hips for support. **Inhale** and lengthen through the body. As you **exhale**, split the legs evenly away from your starting position.* **Inhale** to bring them back to the start and then **exhale** to change sides.

Other considerations:

Avoid sitting heavily into your hands.

Focus on the leg that is moving away from you and keep the knees straight.

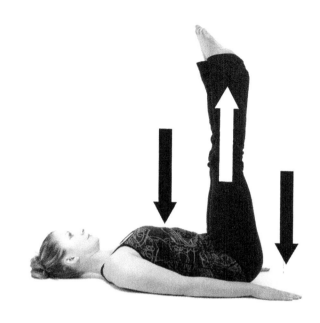

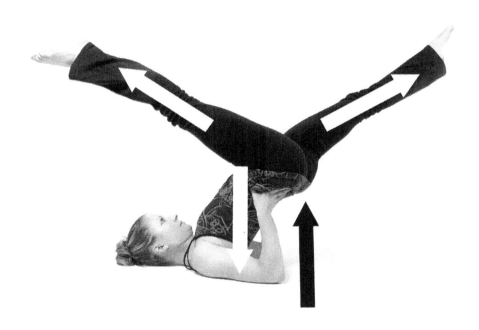

Bicycle
(Advanced)

AIM: To lengthen the hip flexors and strengthen the buttocks, hamstrings and abdominals.

Opposition:

↑ UP: 1 & 2. Maintain a sense of lift through the hips and length through the legs.

↓ DOWN: 1 & 2. Maintain a strong connection between the backs of the arms and the floor.

Directions:

From **Scissors**, **inhale** and lengthen through the body. As you **exhale**, split the legs evenly away from your starting position.* **Inhale** and bend the knee of the leg that is further away from you. Swap the legs over and **exhale** as you straighten the bent leg as it comes toward you and bend the leg that is moving away from you. Keep changing sides and then try reversing it.

Other considerations:

Avoid sitting heavily into your hands.

*Focus on the leg that is moving away from you.

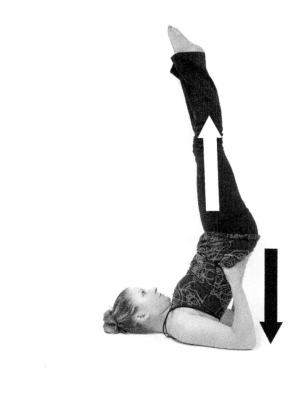

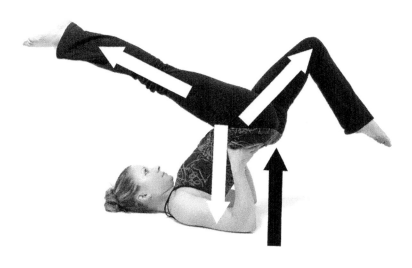

Spine Stretch

AIM: To lengthen the spine and hamstrings.

Opposition:

↑ UP: 1 & 2. Lengthen out through the crown of the head.

↓ DOWN: 1 & 2. Maintain a sense of heaviness through the pelvis.

Other (energy): Lengthen out through the heels and draw in through the abdominals and lower ribcage. Send the arms away *in opposition* to the abdominals.

Directions:

Sit with a straight spine, with your legs out straight in front of you, hip distance apart.* Send the heels away and the toes to the ceiling and the arms out in front of you, slightly above the collarbones. **Inhale** and lengthen through the spine and legs. As you **exhale,** roll the spine forward one bone at a time. Slightly lift the arms. **Inhale** and breathe into the back and sides of your ribcage. **Exhale** to re-stack the spine.

Other considerations:

Keep the shoulders down and the neck long.

* You may feel more comfortable sitting on a block or a pillow.

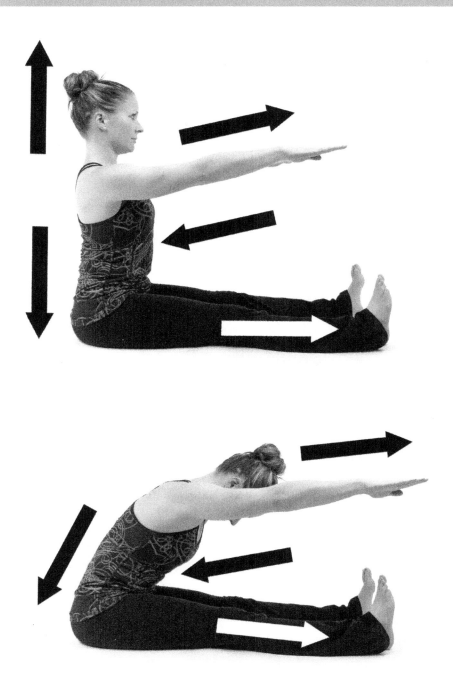

Neck Pull 1

AIM: To strengthen the lower abdominals and lengthen the spine and hamstrings.

Opposition:

↑ UP: 1, 2, 3 & 4. Create a sense of length through the spine.

↓ DOWN: 1, 2, 3 & 4. Maintain a sense of heaviness through your pelvis.

Other (energy): Draw in through the abdominals and lower ribcage and lengthen the legs away through the heels.

Directions:

Sit up straight with your legs out in front of you, shoulder distance apart and stretch the heels away.* Lace your fingers together behind your head, making sure your elbows are in your peripheral vision. **Inhale** and lengthen through the spine. As you **exhale**, lean back slightly moving behind your sitting bones as you do so. **Inhale** and hinge back up to sitting, then as you **exhale**, roll the spine as far forward as you can, pulling the elbows right back.

Other considerations:

Avoid putting pressure on the head and neck as you lean forward.

*You may feel more comfortable sitting on a block or a pillow.

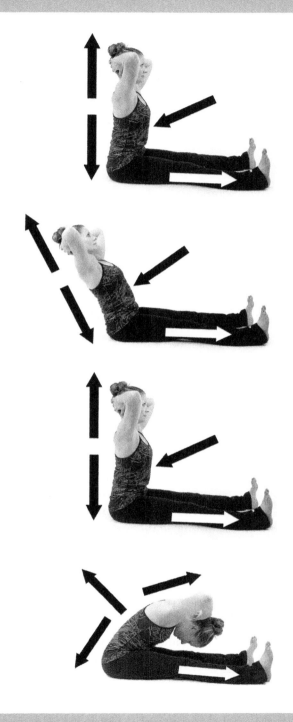

Neck Pull 2
(Advanced)

AIM: To strengthen the abdominals and lengthen the spine and hamstrings. To mobilize the spine.

Opposition:

↑ UP: 1, 2, 3, 4 & 5. Create a sense of length through the spine.

↓ DOWN: 1, 2, 3, 4 & 5. Maintain a sense of heaviness through your pelvis.

Other (energy): Draw in through the abdominals and lower ribcage and lengthen the legs away through the heels.

Directions:

Sit up straight with your legs out in front of you, shoulder distance apart, and stretch the heels away. Lace your fingers together behind your head, making sure your elbows are in your peripheral vision. **Inhale** and lengthen through the spine. As you **exhale**, lean back slightly moving behind your sitting bones as you do so. Continue to roll the spine all the way down to the floor. **Inhale** and start to roll up off your ribcage. **Exhale** and continue to roll all the way up to sitting. **Inhale**, lengthen the spine and then as you **exhale**, roll the spine as far forward as you can, pulling the elbows right back.

Other considerations:

Avoid putting pressure on the head and neck as you lean forward. Try to limit the amount that your legs slide as you roll back and up. Stretch through the knees.

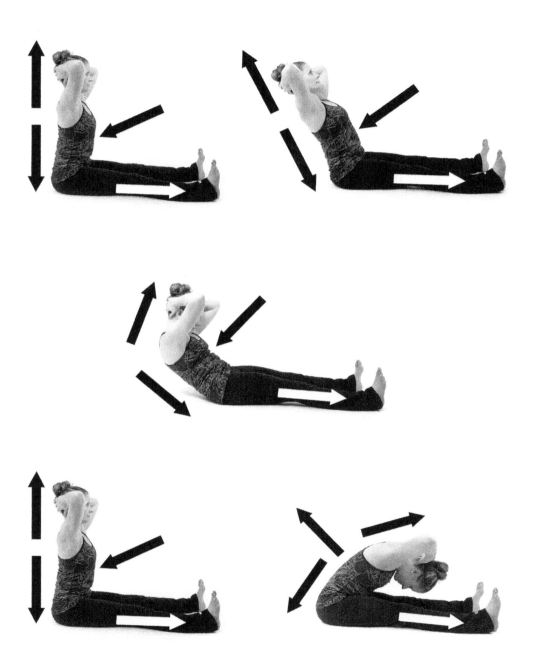

Rocking
(Advanced)

AIM: To stretch the shoulders, abdominals and quadriceps. To strengthen the buttocks.

Opposition:

↑ UP: 1 & 2. Press the feet up and away into the hands.

↓ DOWN: 1 & 2. Create a strong sense of connection through the pelvis.

Other (energy): Lengthen the spine and the crown of the head away from the quadriceps *in opposition.*

Directions:

Lie on your front and bend your knees. Reach back with your hands and grab your feet. **Inhale** to lengthen through the body. As you **exhale**, lift the upper body and the thighs away from the floor by squeezing the buttocks. Press your feet into your hands and your hands into your feet. YOU MAY JUST LOWER BACK DOWN HERE as you **inhale**.

If you wish to advance further, from the lift **inhale** to prepare and as you **exhale**, pull your legs higher to tip your body forward toward the chest and then **inhale** to press the feet away, pulling your body back toward your thighs in a rocking motion.

Other considerations:

Keep the shoulders down and the neck long.

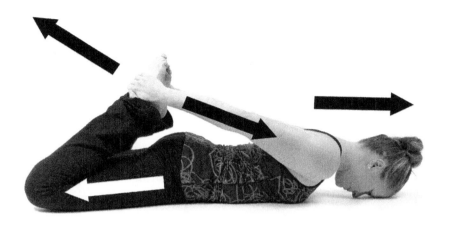

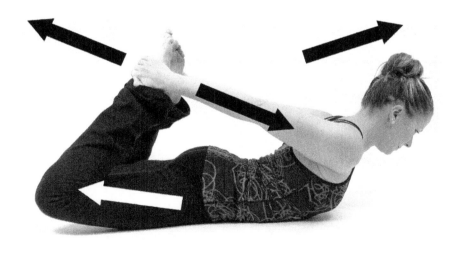

Control and Balance
(Advanced)

AIM: To strengthen the buttocks, lengthen the hamstrings and improve balance.

Opposition:

↑ UP: Lengthen out through the top leg to create lift in the whole body. Stretch the spine.

↓ DOWN: Lengthen out through other leg to keep the body balance on the shoulders.

Directions:

From **The Jack Knife**, carefully move your arms from by your sides to over your head and off the floor. **Inhale** to prepare; as you **exhale**, lower one leg into your hands and then pull the legs away from each other. **Inhale** to swap them over and then exhale to stretch.

Other considerations:

Avoid balancing on your head and neck.

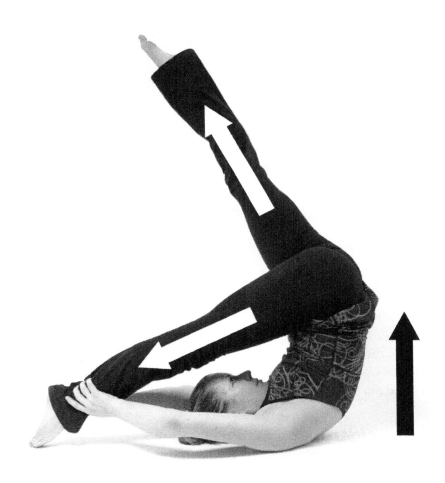

The Roll Down

AIM: To mobilize the spine.

Opposition:

↑ UP: 1. Lengthen out through the crown of the head.

2 & 3. Create a sense of lift through the ribcage.

↓ DOWN: Create a strong sense of connection through the feet.

Directions:

Stand tall with your feet perfectly balanced between the base of the big toes, the base of the little toes and the center of your heels. **Inhale** and lengthen up. As you **exhale**, carefully peel the bones of your spine down one at a time until your shoulders are level with your hips. Allow the arms to hang. **Inhale** and breathe into the back and sides of your ribcage. **Exhale** to roll the spine back up.

Other considerations:

Avoid leaning into your heels as you roll down. *You should feel as if you are laying your spine on to the strong support of your abdominals.*

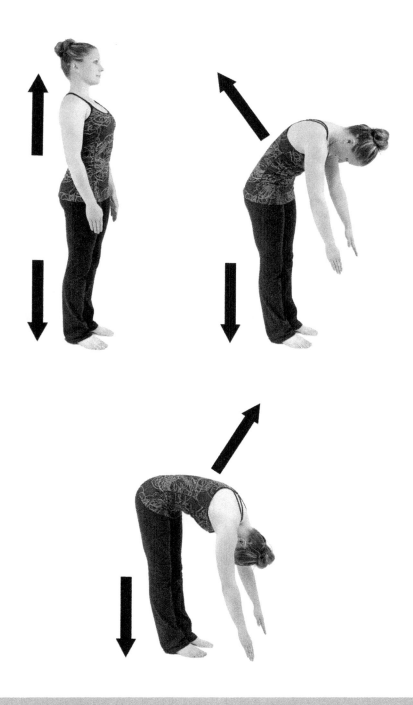

The Workouts

Beginners Pilates

1. The Relaxation Position

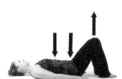

2. Single Knee Fold

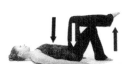

3. Double Knee Fold

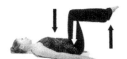

4. Toe Taps 1

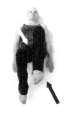

5. Spine Curls

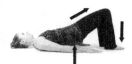

6. Spine Curls with Arms

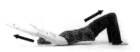

7. Hamstring Stretch 1

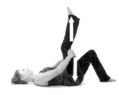

8. Curl Up 1

9. One Hundred 1

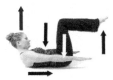

10. Single Leg Stretch

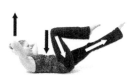

11. Double Leg Stretch 1

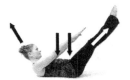

12.Sitting

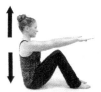

13. Half Roll Back / 'C' Curve

14. The Roll Back 1

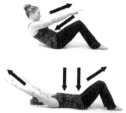

15. The Hip Lift/ The Roll Over 1

16. Upper Back Extension 1

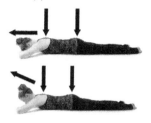

17. Oyster/Side Lying Legs 1

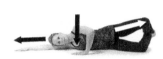

18. Mermaid 1

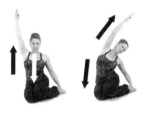

19. Rotation 1

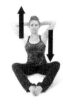
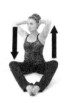

20. Cat

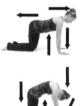

21. Table Top 1

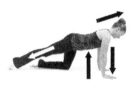

22. Spine Stretch

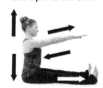
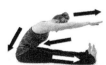

23. The Roll Down

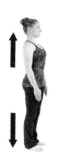
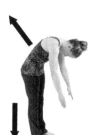
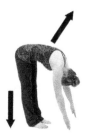

Intermediate Pilates

1. The Relaxation Position
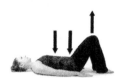

2. Single Knee Fold
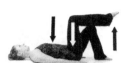

3. Double Knee Fold
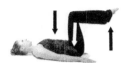

4. The Dying Bug/Toe Taps 2
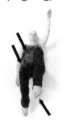

5. Spine Curl
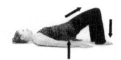

6. Spine Curls with Arms
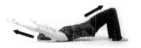

7. Hamstring Stretch 2
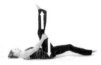

8. Curl Up 2
(with Single Knee Fold)

9. One Hundred 2
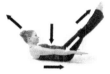

10. Single Leg Stretch 2
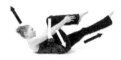

11. Double Leg Stretch 1
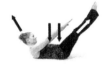

12. The Roll Back 2
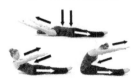

13. The Roll Over 2
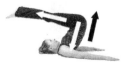

14. Upper Back Extension 2
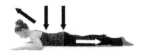

15. Cobra /
Upper Back Extension 3
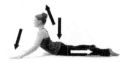

16. Side Lying Legs 2
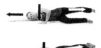

17. Mermaid 1
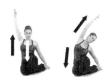

18. Mermaid 2 / Side Hip Lift
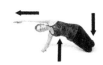

19. Rotation 2

20. Cat
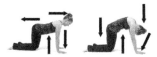

21. Superman/Table Top 2
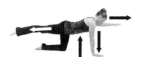

22. Leg Pull Front 1
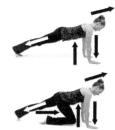

23. Leg Pull Back 1
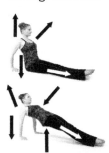

24. Leg Pull Back 2
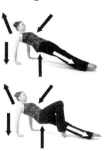

25. Spine Stretch
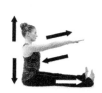

26. Neck Pull 1
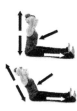

27. The Roll Down
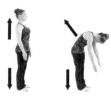

Advanced Pilates

1. The Relaxation Position

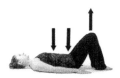

2. Single Knee Fold

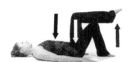

3. Double Knee Fold

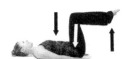

4. The Dying Bug/Toe Taps 2

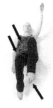

5. Spine Curls with Arms

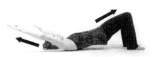

6. Hamstring Stretch

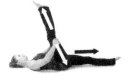

7. Curl Up 3 (with Double Knee Fold)

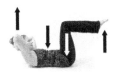

8. Single Leg Stretch 2

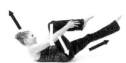

9. Double Leg Stretch 2

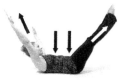

10. The Roll Back 2

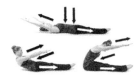

11. The Roll Over 2

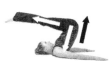

12. Cobra / Back Extension 3

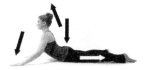

13. Swan Dive 1 / Upper Back Extension 4

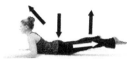

14. Swan Dive 2

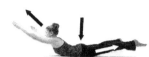

15. Side Lying Legs 3

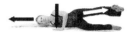
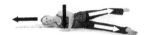

16. Side Lying Legs 4

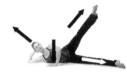

17. Side Lying Legs 5

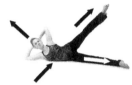

18. Side Twist 1 / Mermaid 3

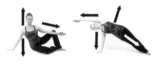

19. Side Twist 2 / Mermaid 4

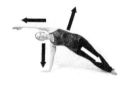

20. The Saw/Rotation 3

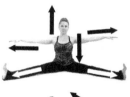
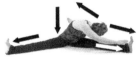

21. Cat

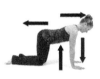
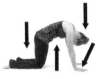

22. Superman / Table Top 2

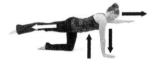

23. Leg Pull Front 2

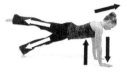

24. Leg Pull Back 3

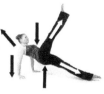

25. The Jack Knife

26. Scissors

27. Bicycle

28. Spine Stretch

29. Neck Pull 2

30. Rocking

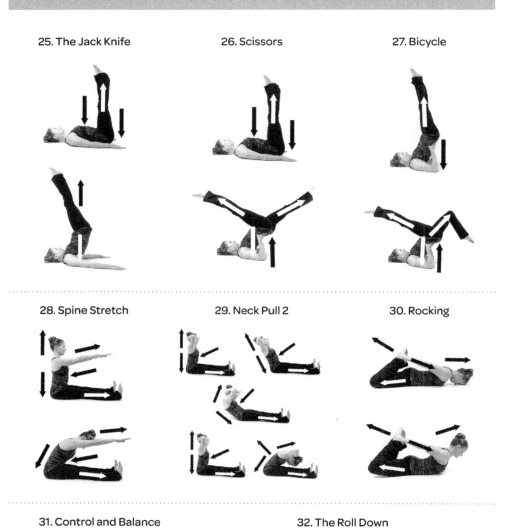

31. Control and Balance

32. The Roll Down

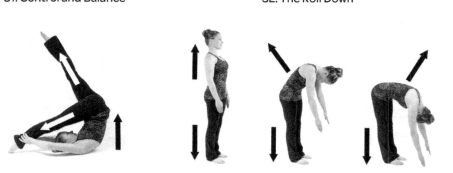

Yoga

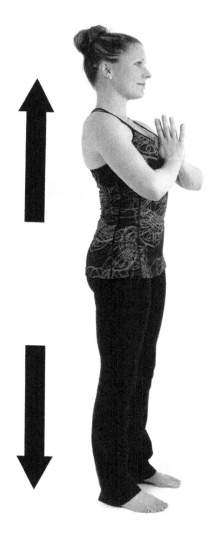

Sukhasana / Easy Pose

AIM: To create mental and physical balance.

Opposition:

↑ UP: Create a sense of length out through the crown of the head.

↓ DOWN: Maintain a sense of heaviness through the pelvis.

Directions:

Sit with your legs crossed and the backs of your hand on the insides of your knees.*
If it feels right to do so, connect your thumb to one of your fingers in a *mudra*. Focus
on your breath. Send the **inhale** deep into the abdomen so that the belly expands.
As you **exhale,** focus on the *opposition* in your spine and notice how the belly and
ribcage draws back in toward your spine.

Other considerations:

Avoid taking tension into the legs; let the knees drop out to the sides.

Sitting on a block or pillow may help you to be more comfortable.

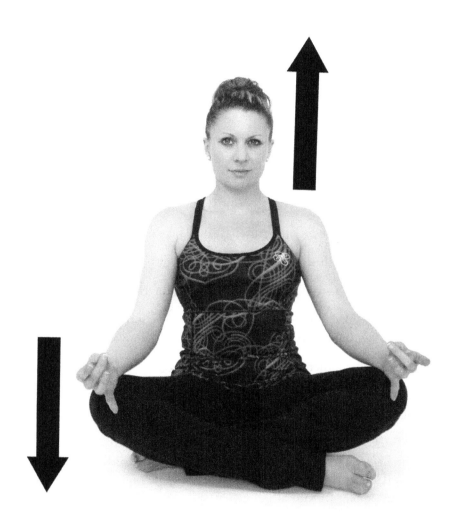

Dwi Pada Pitham / Shoulder Bridge

AIM: To mobilize the spine and create space in the front of the hips. To strengthen the buttocks.

Opposition:

↑ UP: 1. Create a sense of lightness at the knees.

               2. Squeeze the buttocks to lift.

↓ DOWN: 1. Create a strong connection between the ribcage and the floor.

               1 & 2. Maintain a balanced and positive connection between the feet and the floor, particularly the base of the big toe.

OTHER (energy): Lengthen the knees away from you as you lift.

Directions:

Lie on your back with the knees bent and the fingertips just touching the heels. **Inhale** to the back and sides of the ribcage to prepare. **Exhale** and roll the pelvis until the back flattens. Keep rolling and lifting the spine one bone at a time for the duration of the exhale. **Inhale** at the top of the range. **Exhale** and roll the spine back down to the start.

Other considerations:

Avoid lifting the ribcage as you lift up and keep the back of the neck long.

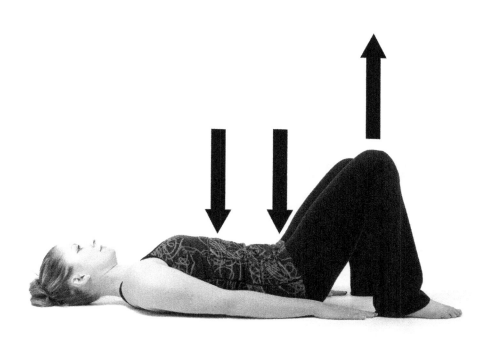

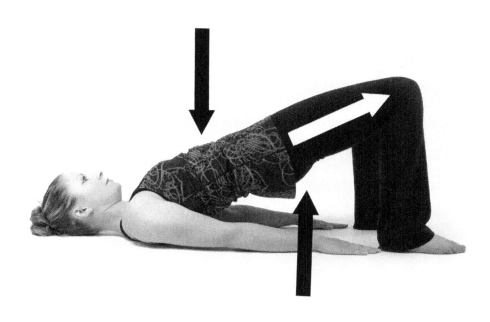

Apanasana / Wind Relieving Pose

AIM: To release tension in the lower back and to stimulate peristalsis.

Opposition:

↑ UP: Create a sense of lightness at the knees.

↓ DOWN: Maintain a sense of heaviness through the pelvis and a strong connection between the ribcage and the floor.

Directions:

Lie on your back and pull your knees in toward your chest. Place your hands on your knees. **Inhale** and gently push the knees away from you. As you **exhale,** circle the legs out to the sides and in toward your abdomen. Keep circling and breathing, changing direction when you feel ready.

Other considerations:

Keep the back of the neck long and the chin down.

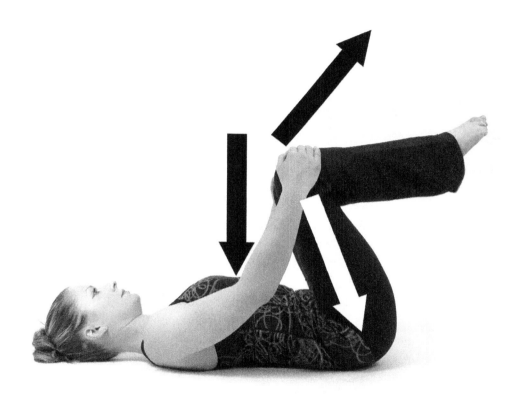

Bidalasana / Cat / Cow

AIM: To mobilize the whole spine and stretch and strengthen the lower abdominals. To strengthen the upper back muscles.

Opposition:

↑ UP: 1 & 2. Create a sense of lift through the bottom of the ribcage and lower abdominals.

3. Send the tailbone up and away from the crown of the head.

↓ DOWN: 1, 2 & 3. Maintain a strong connection through the whole of the hand.

2. Drop the head and tailbone down to the floor.

Other (energy):

Send the breastbone forward and up *in opposition* to the tailbone.

Directions:

Position your body in a four-point kneeling position, with the hands* directly underneath the shoulders and the knees directly underneath the hips. Lengthen the spine. **Inhale**; then as you **exhale**, tuck the buttocks under, sending your spine to the ceiling and your head and tailbone to the floor. DO NOT SQUEEZE YOUR BUTTOCKS AND LEGS. Hold the position and take a full **inhale** to the back and sides of your ribcage. **Exhale** to lengthen out of the position. As you **inhale**, send the breastbone forward and the tailbone upward. **Exhale** to pull yourself back into the **Cat**.

Other considerations:

Keep the shoulders down and the neck long. Keep the ribcage and abdominals drawn in toward the spine.

If this makes your wrists uncomfortable, try balancing on fists.

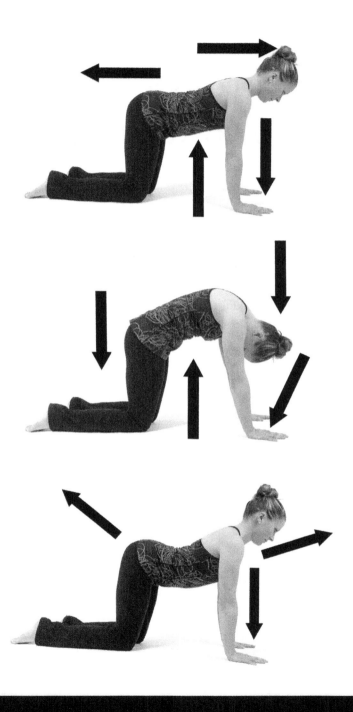

Adho Mukha Svanasana / Downward Dog

AIM: To revitalize the whole body. To stretch the hamstrings and spine. To strengthen the arms.

Opposition:

↑ UP: Create a sense of lift from the tailbone.

↓ DOWN: Maintain a strong sense of connection through the hands and lengthen the heels toward the floor.

Directions:

From **Cat/Cow,** tuck the toes under and send the tailbone to the ceiling, stretching the legs out straight* so that you are in an inverted 'V' position. Hold the pose for a count of three full **inhales** and **exhales**. Every time you **inhale**, focus on creating space in the back; every time you **exhale**, focus on length as you lift your hips to the ceiling and send your heels to the floor. Come out of the pose by either returning to **Cat/Cow** or walking the hands backward into a **standing forward bend**.

Other considerations:

If the backs of your legs are tight, keep the knees slightly bent so that you can maintain a straight spine.

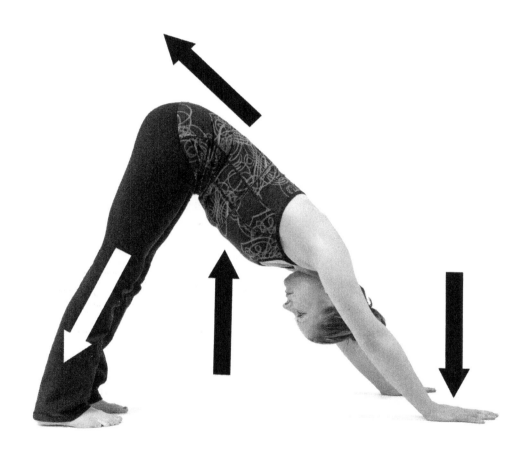

Uttanasana / Standing Forward Bend

AIM: To lengthen the backs of the legs and the spine.

Opposition:

↑ UP: 1 & 2. Create a sense of length through the back of the legs and lift through the ribcage.

↓ DOWN: 1 & 2. Maintain a strong sense of connection through the feet.

2. Allow the head to drop heavily toward the floor.

Other (energy): Send the breastbone and tailbone away from each other *in opposition.*

Directions:

From either **Downward Dog** or **Mountain Pose**, bring the body into a forward bend position. You can hold the pose here for three breaths, holding your elbows or letting the arms hang. Focus on taking the **inhale** into the back and sides of your ribcage. **Exhale** and lengthen through the legs and spine. Alternatively, **inhale** and take your hands on to either your lower or upper legs. Send the breastbone forward and lengthen the spine. **Exhale** and drop the body forward back into **Standing Forward Bend**. Repeat.

Other considerations:

Avoid shortening the back of your neck when you lift up.

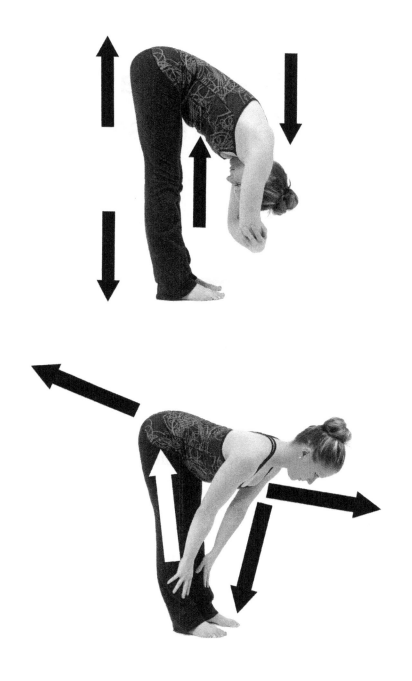

Utkatasana / Fierce Pose

AIM: To strengthen the legs and back.

Opposition:

↑ UP: Lengthen out through the arms and create a sense of lift through the ribs.

↓ DOWN: Maintain a positive connection through the feet and lengthen the tailbone away from the crown of the head.

Directions:

From **Mountain Pose** or **Standing Forward Bend**, drop the hips down and bend your knees. Send the arms away to a 45 degree and stretch the tailbone away from you.* Hold the pose and **inhale** and **exhale** fully three times. Return to your starting position.

Other considerations:

Avoid shortening the back of the neck and keep the shoulders down.

Keep the arms either shoulder distance apart or bring the palms together, join the fingers and point the index fingers away from you.

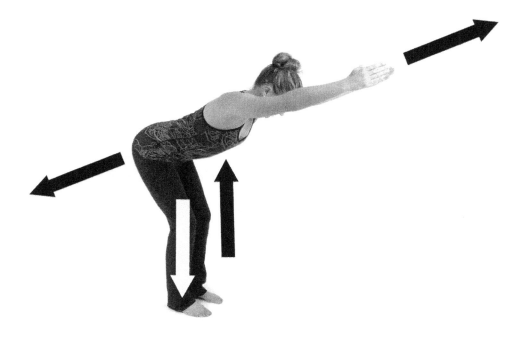

Tadasana / Mountain Pose

AIM: To develop physical and mental balance. To improve standing posture.

Opposition:

↑ UP: Lengthen out through the crown of the head.

↓ DOWN: Maintain a strong sense of connection through the feet.

Directions:

Stand with your feet hip distance apart and slightly turned out.* Balance your feet between the base of your big toes, the base of the little toes and the center of the back of the heels. If you would like to, bring the palms together in front of your breastbone with the thumbs touching your heart chakra (the center of the breastbone) or leave the arms hanging by your sides. If you would like to, close your eyes. Focus on your breathing. **Inhale** into the abdomen, allowing the belly and ribcage to expand. As you **exhale**, feel the belly draw back in, followed by the ribcage.

This is not the traditional position for the feet in yoga, but it is biomechanically more efficient.

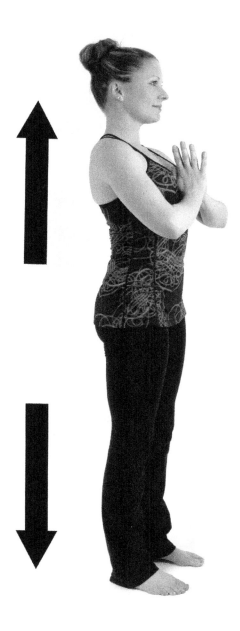

High Lunge

AIM: To lengthen hip flexors and create space through the whole body.

Opposition:

↑ UP: Send the breastbone forward and up.

↓ DOWN: Lengthen the heel of the back leg away and sink the hips toward the floor.

Directions:

From **Uttanasana**, place your hands either side of your feet and **inhale** and step back with one leg. **Exhale** and stretch through the whole body. **Inhale** and send the breastbone forward so that your upper spine is in slight extension. Hold the posture and breathe steadily until you are ready to change sides.

Other considerations:

Keep the back of the neck long and the shoulders relaxed.

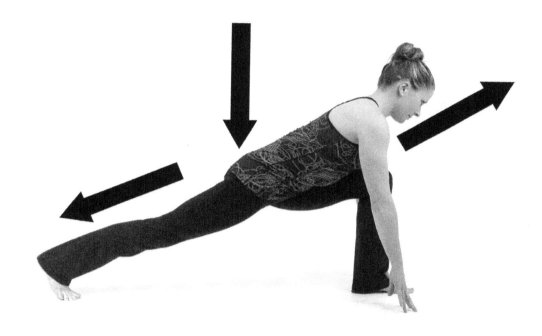

High Plank

AIM: To create strength in the abdominals and arms. To focus the mind and balance the whole body.

Opposition:

↑ UP: Create a sense of lift from the bottom of the ribcage.

↓ DOWN: Maintain a firm connection between the hands and the floor.

Other (energy): Create a sense of *opposition* between the heels and the crown of the head.

Directions:

From **High Lunge**, place your hands either side of your feet and **inhale** and step back with your other leg. **Exhale** and stretch through the whole body. Hold the posture and breathe steadily until you are ready to move on.

Other considerations:

Keep the back of the neck long and the shoulders relaxed.

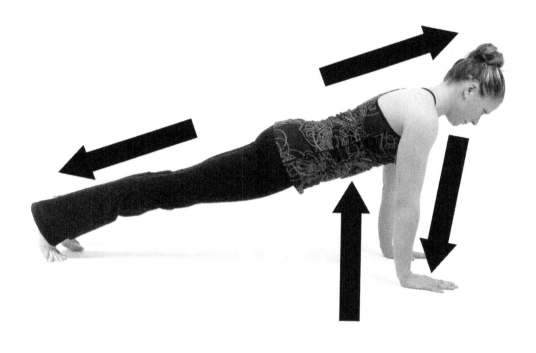

Half Plank

AIM: To provide a comfortable transition between plank postures and prone postures.

Opposition:

↑ UP: Create a sense of lift from the bottom of the ribcage.

↓ DOWN: Maintain a strong connection between the hands and the floor.

Other (energy): Lengthen the crown of the head away from the tailbone.

Directions:

To transition from **High Plank**, **inhale** and take the knees to the floor and lengthen the lower legs and feet so that they are flat on the floor. Keep your upper body weight over your hands before you **exhale** and lower into **Cobra**.

Other considerations:

Keep the back of the neck long and the shoulders relaxed.

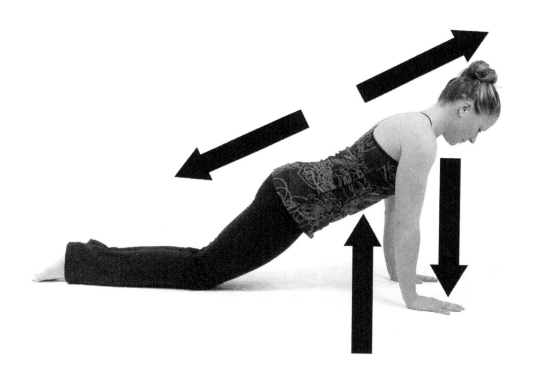

Chaturanga / 4 Limbed Staff Pose

AIM: To lengthen whole body and to strengthen the arms.

Opposition:

↑ UP: Maintain a sense of lift from the bottom of the ribcage and from the hips.

↓ DOWN: Maintain a strong connection between the hands and the floor.

Other (energy): Lengthen the legs away from the crown of the head.

Directions:

From **High Plank, inhale** and lengthen through the whole body. **Exhale** and slowly lower your whole body so that it hovers just off the floor. **Inhale** and transition to **Upward Facing Dog** by rolling over your toes and sliding the body forward and up.

Other considerations:

Keep the back of the neck long and the shoulders relaxed.

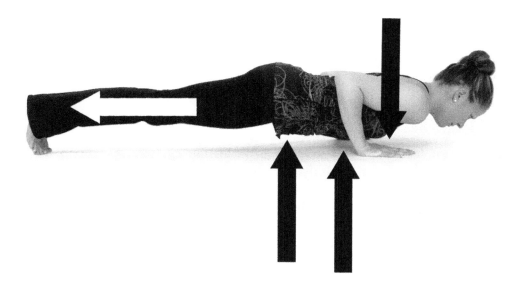

Cobra

AIM: To gently stretch the front of the shoulders and extend the upper spine.

Opposition:

Other (energy): Send the elbows toward the ankles and lengthen the breastbone away *in opposition.*

Directions:

Lie on your front with your toes together and your heels dropped apart. Relax the buttocks. Place your hands underneath your shoulders so that your elbows are pointing up and the arms are close to your body. **Exhale** and settle the front of your body on to the floor. As you **inhale**, peel your upper body up off the floor without putting any pressure through your hands. Send the elbows away from your ears. **Exhale** to lower to the floor and repeat.

Other considerations:

Keep the back of the neck long and the shoulders relaxed. Avoid gripping the buttocks and keep the lower back long.

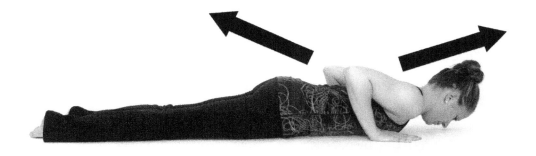

Urdhva Mukha Svanasana / Upward Facing Dog
(Advanced)

AIM: To lengthen hip flexors, extend the upper spine and strengthen the arms.

Opposition:

↑ UP: Send the breastbone forward and up.

↓ DOWN: Maintain a strong connection between the hands and the floor.

Other (energy): Lengthen the legs away from the crown of the head.

Directions:

From **4 Limbed Staff Pose, exhale** and stretch through the whole body. **Inhale** and send the breastbone forward so that your upper spine is in slight extension. **Exhale** and send the body backward into **Downward Facing Dog**.

Other considerations:

Keep the back of the neck long and the shoulders relaxed.

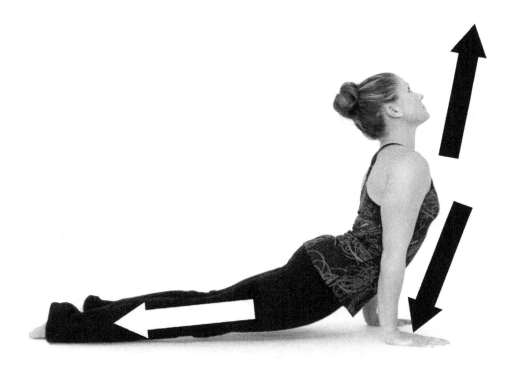

Purvottanasana / Inclined Plank Pose

AIM: To strengthen the buttocks and arms. To lengthen the whole body.

Opposition:

↑ UP: Create a strong sense of lift from underneath the buttocks.

↓ DOWN: Maintain a strong connection between the hands and the floor. Keep the lower ribcage drawn in.

Other (energy): Lengthen the legs away from the crown of the head.

Directions:

Sit tall with the legs straight out in front of you and the hands behind you. Your fingers should be pointing toward the feet, elbows bent, the body slightly leaning backwards. **Inhale** and lengthen through the spine. As you **exhale**, squeeze the buttocks and lift your hips off the floor, lengthening through the whole body. **Inhale** and hold the posture before **exhaling** to lower slowly.

Other considerations:

Avoid 'throwing' the head backwards. Your eyeline should be directed away at a 45 degree angle. Stretch through the knees.

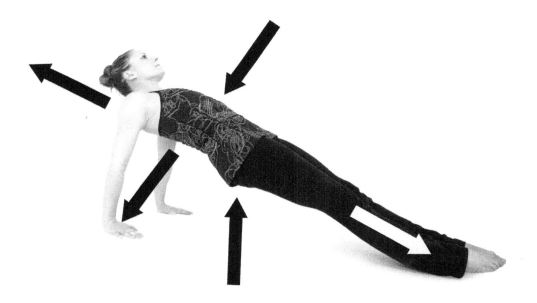

Paschimottanasana / Seated Forward Bend

AIM: To lengthen the whole of the back of the body.

Opposition:

↓ **DOWN:**   Maintain a strong connection between the pelvis and the floor. Allow the head to hang heavily.

Other (energy): Lengthen the legs and sitting bones away from each other.

Directions:

Sit tall with the legs straight out in front of you and the hands on your legs.* **Inhale** and lengthen through the spine. As you **exhale**, relax your upper body forward to a comfortable position. Hold the posture and breathe steadily until you are ready to come out.

Other considerations:

Relax your shoulders.

Sitting on a small pillow or block may help you feel more comfortable.

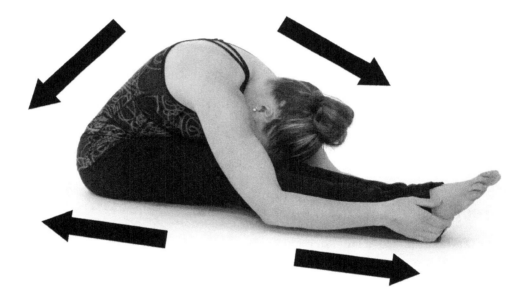

Virabhadrasana 1 / Warrior 1

AIM: To strengthen and lengthen the legs and trunk.

Opposition:

↑ UP: 1. Create a strong sense of lift from the arms.

2. Create a strong sense of lift from the arms and breastbone.

↓ DOWN: 1 & 2. Maintain a positive connection between the feet and the floor. Lengthen through the back leg.

Other (energy): Send the front knee away from the back leg (in line with your second toe).

Directions:

From **Tadasana**, take a large step back and position your foot at a 45 degree angle (pointing toward the front foot). Position your body facing toward your front leg. **Inhale** and lift both of your arms up above your head, joining them together if it feels comfortable. **Exhale** and bend your front leg, sending the knee in the same direction as the second toe.* **Inhale**; lengthen through the whole body and **exhale** to sink into the posture a little more deeply.

Other considerations:

Keep the shoulders down and the spine long. Keep both feet firmly in contact with the floor. Avoid gripping with your toes.

Avoid sending the knee over the second toe.

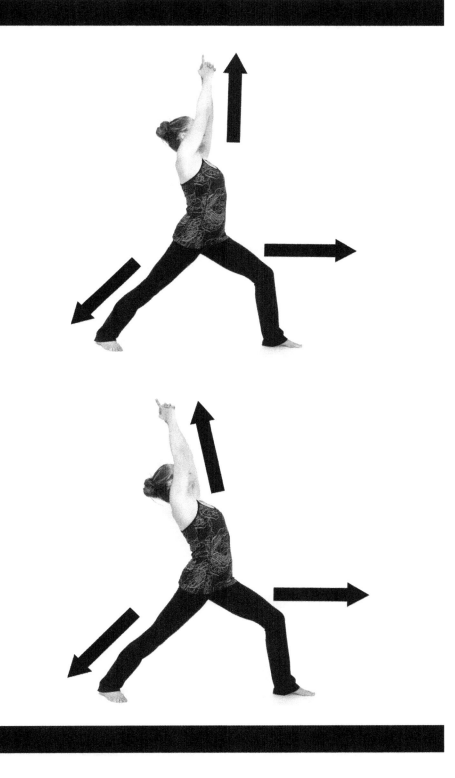

█████████████████████████████████████

Virabhadrasana / Warrior 2

AIM: To strengthen and lengthen the legs and trunk.

Opposition:

↑ UP: Lengthen out through the crown of the head.

↓ DOWN: Maintain length through the back leg and a strong connection between the feet and the floor.

Other (energy): Send the front knee away from the back leg (in line with your second toe). Stretch the arms away from each other.

Directions:

From **Warrior 1**, **inhale** and lengthen up. **Exhale** and bring the arms down so that they are in line with the collarbones and sink a little deeper into the posture. Hold and breathe steadily until you are ready to come out.

Other considerations:

Keep the shoulders down and the spine long. Keep both feet firmly in contact with the floor. Avoid gripping with your toes.

Avoid sending the knee over the second toe.

█████████████████████████████████████

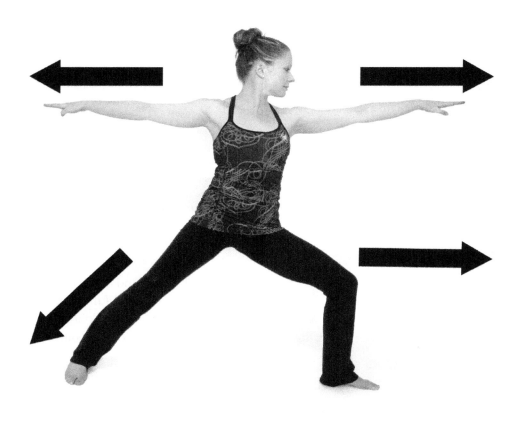

Trikonasana / Triangle Pose

AIM: To strengthen and lengthen the legs and trunk. To lengthen the waistline.

Opposition:

↑ UP: Lengthen out through the top arm and the ribs.

↓ DOWN: Maintain length through the legs and a strong connection between the feet and the floor. Lengthen the bottom arm toward the floor.

Directions:

From **Warrior 2, inhale** and straighten the front leg. **Exhale** and lower your front arm so that the back of your hand is on the inside of your front leg.* Lift up the back arm until it is vertical with the palm forward. Turn your head to look at your top hand. Hold the posture and breathe steadily until you are ready to come out.

Other considerations:

Keep the shoulders down and the spine long. Keep both feet firmly in contact with the floor. Avoid gripping with your toes.

Where you put your hand is determined by your ability to maintain a straight spine.

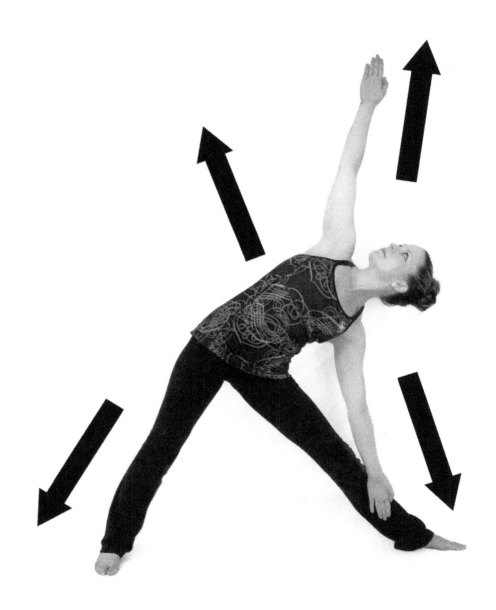

Utthita Parsvakonasana / Extended Side Angle
(Advanced)

AIM: To strengthen and lengthen the legs and trunk. To lengthen the waistline.

Opposition:

↑ UP: Lengthen out through the top arm and the ribs.

↓ DOWN: Maintain length through the legs and a strong connection between the feet and the floor. Create a strong connection between the bent elbow and your thigh.

Directions:

From **Triangle Pose**, **inhale** and lift out into **Warrior 2**; as you **exhale**, bend the front knee and place your elbow on the thigh. Stretch the free arm over your head, lengthening the waist and lifting the ribs. Breathe steadily and hold the posture until you are ready to come out.

Other considerations:

Keep the shoulders down and the spine long. Keep both feet firmly in contact with the floor. Avoid gripping with your toes.

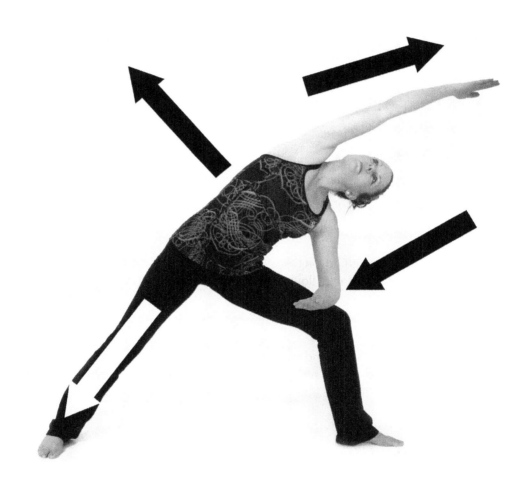

Prasarita Padottanasana / Wide Legged Forward Bend
(Advanced)

AIM: To lengthen the legs and the spine.

Opposition:

↑ UP: Create a sense of lift from the tailbone.

↓ DOWN: Maintain length through the legs and a strong connection between the feet and the floor. Allow the head to drop heavily toward the floor.

Directions:

Stand with the feet wide apart and your body facing forward in the same direction as both feet. **Inhale** and lengthen through the spine. **Exhale** and carefully roll the body forward until you are touching the floor with your hands, arms or arms and head. Hold the posture and breathe steadily until you are ready to come out.

Other considerations:

Relax your head and neck. Keep both feet firmly in contact with the floor. Avoid gripping with your toes.

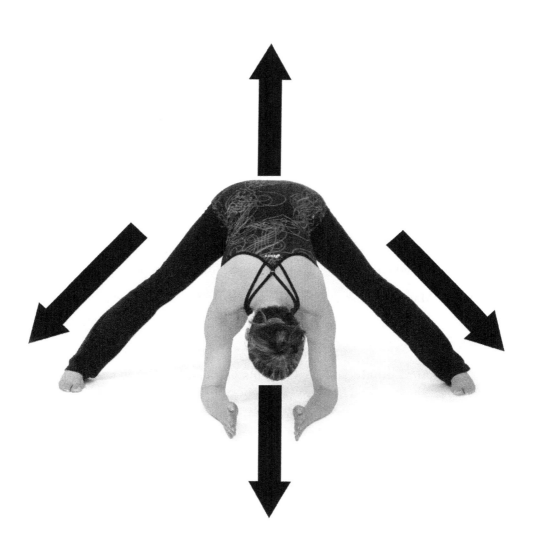

Urdhva Hastasana / Upward Salute

AIM: To lengthen and extend the spine.

Opposition:

↑ UP: Lengthen out through the arms and the breastbone.

↓ DOWN: Maintain a strong sense of connection through the feet.

Directions:

From **Tadasana**, **inhale** and lift the arms up, joining them together if it feels comfortable. Slightly lift the breastbone, squeeze the buttocks and send the hips forward. **Exhale** to lower back down.

Other considerations:

Avoid collapsing into the lower back and lengthen the legs. Keep the back of the neck long.

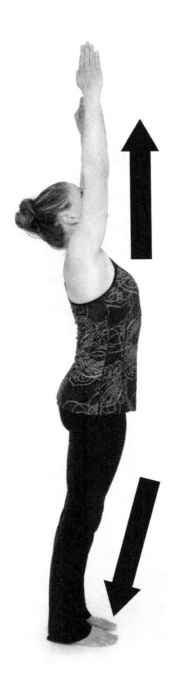

Vrksasana / Tree Pose
(Advanced)

AIM: To create stillness and balance in mind and body.

Opposition:

↑ UP: 1. Lengthen out through the crown of the head.

2. Lengthen out through the crown of the head and the arms.

↓ DOWN: 1 & 2. Maintain length through the legs and a strong connection between the feet and the floor.

Directions:

From **Tadasana**, **inhale** and lengthen the spine. As you **exhale**, balance on one leg and position/press the free leg/foot on to somewhere comfortable on the inside of your standing leg. If you are stretching the arms up, **inhale** and lengthen. Focus your gaze on an immovable spot in front of you. Hold the posture and breathe steadily until you are ready to change sides.

Other considerations:

Keep the shoulders down and the spine long. Keep the foot firmly in contact with the floor. Avoid gripping with your toes.

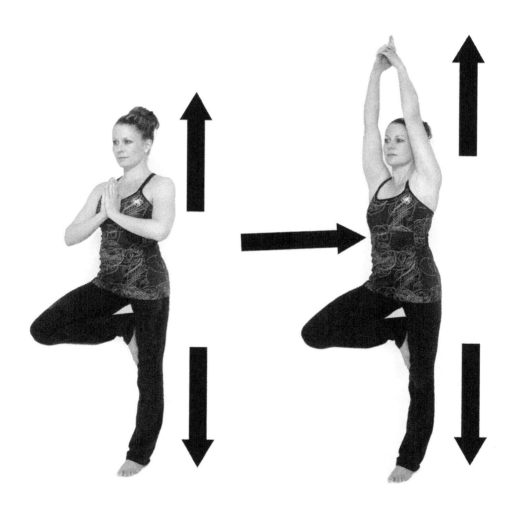

Natarajasana / Dancer Pose
(Advanced)

AIM: To strengthen the legs and buttocks. To stretch the quadriceps and hip flexors. To improve balance.

Opposition:

↑ UP: 1 & 2. Lengthen out through the crown of the head.

↓ DOWN: 1 & 2. Lengthen the thigh toward the floor. Maintain length through the legs and a strong connection between the feet and the floor.

Other (energy): Lengthen the arms and thigh away from each other.

Directions:

From **Tadasana, inhale** and lengthen the spine. As you **exhale**, balance on one leg and bring the free foot toward your buttock. Hold the foot. **Inhale**; as you **exhale**, fix your eyes on an immovable spot in front of you and tip the body forward, stretching the free arm away from you and lifting the other leg up behind you. Hold the posture and breathe steadily until you are ready to come out and change sides.

Other considerations:

Keep the shoulders down and the spine long. Keep the foot firmly in contact with the floor. Avoid gripping with your toes.

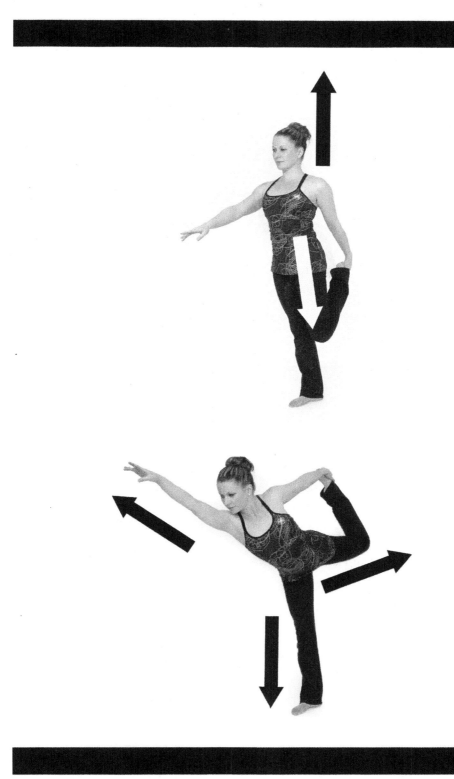

Utthita Hasta Padangusthasana / Extended Hand to Big Toe Pose
(Advanced)

AIM: To strengthen the legs and buttocks. To stretch and strengthen the quadriceps and hip flexors. To improve balance.

Opposition:

↑ UP: 1 & 2. Lengthen out through the crown of the head.

↓ DOWN: 1 & 2. Maintain length through the standing leg and a strong sense of connection between the foot and the floor.

Directions:

From **Tadasana, inhale** and lengthen the spine. As you **exhale**, balance on one leg and bring the free foot into your hand. Grasp your big toe.* **Inhale**; as you **exhale**, fix your eyes on an immovable spot in front of you and stretch the leg out in front of you (or to the side of you). Hold the posture and breathe steadily until you are ready to come out and change sides.

Other considerations:

Keep the shoulders down and the spine long. Keep the foot firmly in contact with the floor. Avoid gripping with your toes.

If the backs of your legs are tight, hold the back of the thigh instead of the toe.

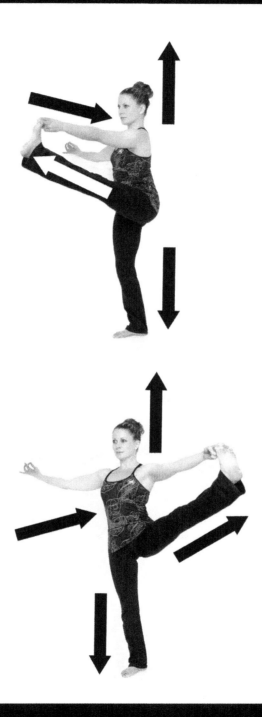

Surya Namaskara / Sun Salutation

(Beginners)

1.

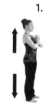

2.

3.

4.

5.

6.

7.

8.

9.

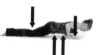

10.

11.

12.

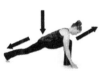

13.

14.

15.

Surya Namaskara / Sun Salutation

(Advanced)

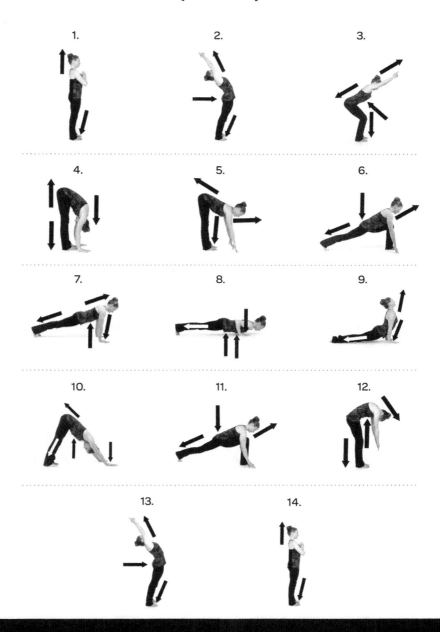

Beginners Practice

1. Sukhasana / Easy Pose

2. Dwi Pada Pitham / Shoulder Bridge

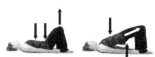

3. Apanasana / Wind Relieving Pose

4. Bidalasana / Cat / Cow

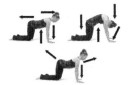

5. Adho Mukha Svanasana / Downward Dog

6. Uttanasana / Standing Forward Bend

7. Tadasana / Mountain Pose

8. Utkatasana / Fierce Pose

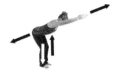

9. Beginners Sun Salutation (See p192)

10. Virabhadrasana 1 / Warrior 1

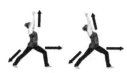

11. Virabhadrasana 2 / Warrior 2

12. Trikonasana / Triangle Pose

13. Purvottanasana / Inclined Plank Pose

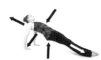

14. Paschimottanasana / Seated Forward Bend

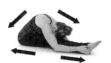

15. Sukhasana / Easy Pose

Advanced Practice

1. Sukhasana / Easy Pose

2. Dwi Pada Pitham / Shoulder Bridge

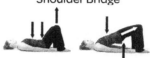

3. Apanasana / Wind Relieving Pose

4. Bidalasana / Cat / Cow

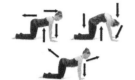

5. Adho Mukha Svanasana / Downward Dog

6. Uttanasana / Standing Forward Bend

7. Advanced Sun Salutation (See p193)

8. Virabhadrasana 1 / Warrior 1

9. Virabhadrasana 2 / Warrior 2

10. Trikonasana / Triangle pose

11. Utthita Parsvakonasana / Extended Side Angle

12. Prasarita Padottanasana / Wide Legged Forward Bend

13. Vrksasana / Tree Pose

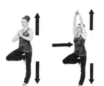

14. Natarajasana / Dancer Pose

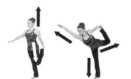

15. Utthita Hasta Padangusthasana / Extended Hand to Big Toe Pose

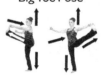

16. Purvottanasana / Inclined Plank Pose

17. Paschimottanasana / Seated Forward Bend

18. Sukhasana / Easy Pose

About the Author

Marie-Claire has worked in the fitness industry since 1998 in a number of different disciplines: gym instructor, personal trainer, swimming teacher, sports massage therapist and so on, but predominantly since 2002 she has worked as a Pilates and Yoga teacher. Other work includes Associate Lecturer at University College Chichester on the Sports Biomechanics program and as a fitness presenter at conventions held around the UK.

Marie-Claire Pilates Studios was founded in 2004 in Southampton. In 2007 she joined forces with a West Sussex based fitness teacher training company called Fitness Inspired Teacher Training (Fitt) and is the sole author and presenter of the Fitt Pilates Teacher Training program/equipment training courses and yoga course tutor. She continues to work alongside Fitt to bring high quality teacher training to the whole of the UK.

In 2012 Marie-Claire headed out to the U.S. to work at a studio in Florida and train alongside those who were educated by Joseph Pilates himself.

Marie-Claire specifically worked with individuals who had injuries, pre- and post-surgery and illnesses such as cancer and multiple sclerosis, dedicating the studio's charity fundraising to the MS Trust after losing a beloved client to the disease.

In 2014 an accident caused so much damage in her own back that she had to move away from teaching every day and sold the studio in 2015. Her new business The Movement Specialist is dedicated to supporting those individuals wishing to advance their careers – either through targeting teacher training in centers, or offering business support and advice. Marie-Claire continues to work privately on a referral basis with people who would like to participate in generalized classes but feel that their physical restrictions (illness/injury) are holding them back. Through educating, understanding, rehabilitating and communicating with their regular teacher, she aims to have **everyone** getting the most out of their Pilates and Yoga classes, including herself.

www.themovementspecialist.co.uk

f   Marie-Claire Pilates and Yoga Specialist

🐦 MCPilatesYoga

📷 themovementspecialist

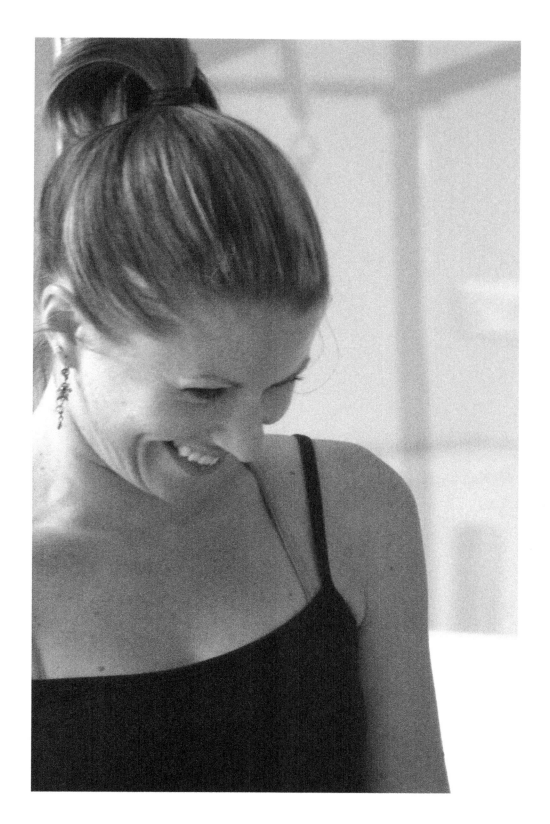